Official Journal of the 'Mediterranean League against Thromboembolic Diseases'

Hæmostasis

International Journal on Haemostasis and Thrombosis Research

AF884761

KARGER

Printed in Italy by CPZ Litografia sas, Costa di Mezzate

Appears bimonthly: 1 volume per year (6 issues)

Guidelines for Authors

Hæmostasis

Submission

Only original papers written in English that communicate novel findings in the field of haemostasis and thrombosis are considered. Both contributions to the basic understanding of these processes and reports on clinical management of disorders in this field are acceptable. Manuscripts can be sent either to the managing editor or to one of the editors as listed in each issue of Haemostasis.
Manuscripts should be submitted in triplicate (with three sets of illustrations of which one is an original), typewritten double-spaced on one side of the paper, with a wide margin.

Conditions

All manuscripts are subject to editorial review. A manuscript is to be considered rejected when an author does not return a revised manuscript within 3 months of receiving the suggestions for revision, unless the author explains further delay. Manuscripts are received with the explicit understanding that they are not under simultaneous consideration by any other publication. Submission of an article for publication implies the transfer of the copyright from the author to the publisher upon acceptance. Accepted papers become the permanent property of 'Haemostasis' and may not be reproduced by any means, in whole or in part, without the written consent of both the author and the publisher. It is the author's responsibility to obtain permission to reproduce illustrations, tables, etc. from other publications.

Arrangement

Title page: The first page of each paper should indicate the title, the authors' names, and the institute where the work was conducted. A short title for use as running head as well as the full address of the author to whom correspondence should be sent are also required.

Full address: The exact postal address complete with postal code must be given at the bottom of the title page. Please also supply phone and fax numbers, as well as your e-mail address.

Key words: For indexing purposes, a list of 3–10 key words in English is essential.

Abstract: Each paper needs an abstract of up to 10 lines.

Small type: Paragraphs which can or must be set in smaller type (case histories, test methods, etc.) should be indicated with a 'p' (petit) in the margin on the left-hand side.

Footnotes: Avoid footnotes. When essential, they are numbered consecutively and typed at the foot of the appropriate page.

Tables and illustrations: Tables and illustrations (both numbered in Arabic numerals) should be prepared on separate sheets. Tables require a heading and figures a legend, also prepared on a separate sheet. For the reproduction of illustrations, only good drawings and original photographs can be accepted; negatives or photocopies cannot be used. Due to technical reasons, figures with a screen background should not be submitted. When possible, group several illustrations on one block for reproduction (max. size 144 × 196 mm) or provide crop marks. On the back of each illustration, indicate its number, the author's name, and 'top' with a soft pencil.

Color illustrations: Up to 6 color illustrations per page can be integrated within the text at the reduced price of CHF 660.– / USD 545.00 per page. Color illustrations are reproduced at the author's expense.

References: In the text identify references by Arabic numerals [in square brackets]. Material submitted for publication but not yet accepted should be noted as 'unpublished data' and not be included in the reference list. The list of references should include only those publications which are cited in the text. Do not alphabetize; number references in the order in which they are first mentioned in the text. The surnames of the authors followed by initials should be given. There should be no punctuation other than a comma to separate the authors. Cite all authors, 'et al' is not sufficient. Abbreviate journal names according to the Index Medicus system. (Also see International Committee of Medical Journal Editors: Uniform requirements for manuscripts submitted to biomedical journals. N Engl J Med 1997;336:309–315.)

(a) Papers published in periodicals: Sun J, Koto H, Chung KF: Interaction of ozone and allergen challenges on bronchial responsiveness and inflammation in sensitised guinea pigs. Int Arch Allergy Immunol 1997;112:191–195.

(b) Monographs: Matthews DE, Farewell VT: Using and Understanding Medical Statistics, ed 3, revised. Basel, Karger, 1996.

(c) Edited books: Parren PWHI, Burton DR: Antibodies against HIV-1 from phage display libraries: Mapping of an immune response and progress towards antiviral immunotherapy; in Capra JD (ed): Antibody Engineering. Chem Immunol. Basel, Karger, 1997, vol 65, pp 18–56.

Page charges

There are no page charges for papers of 6 or fewer printed pages (including tables, illustrations and references). Each additional complete or partial page is charged to the author at CHF 275.– / USD 196.00. The allotted size of a paper is equal to approx. 12 manuscript pages (including tables, illustrations and references).

Galley proofs

Unless indicated otherwise, galley proofs are sent to the first-named author and should be returned with the least possible delay. Alterations made in galley proofs, other than the correction of printer's errors, are charged to the author. No page proofs are supplied.

Reprints

Order forms and a price list are sent with the galley proofs. Orders submitted after the issue is printed are subject to considerably higher prices.

KARGER

Fax + 41 61 306 12 34
E-Mail karger@karger.ch
www.karger.com

The Guidelines for Authors are available at:
www.karger.com/journals/hae/hae_gl.htm

Hæmostasis

General Information

Publication data: 'Haemostasis' is published 6 times a year. Volume 31 with 6 issues appears in 2001.

Subscription rates: Subscriptions run for a full calendar year. Prices are given per volume.
Personal subscription:
Subscription + postage and handling
CHF 322.– + CHF 27.40 Europe
CHF 322.– + CHF 40.80 Overseas
USD 247.50 + USD 27.40
+ online subscription per volume:
CHF 39.– / USD 30.00
(Must be in the name of, billed to, and paid by an individual. Order must be marked 'personal subscription'.)
Institutional subscription:
Subscription + postage and handling
CHF 644.– + CHF 34.20 Europe
CHF 644.– + CHF 46.20 Overseas
USD 495.00 + USD 34.20
+ online subscription per volume:
CHF 58.– / USD 45.00
Airmail postage: CHF 36.–, USD 30.00.
(Extra per volume.)
Discount subscription prices:
Gesellschaft für Thrombose- und Haemostase-Forschung;
International Society of Haematology.

Microforms: Please direct all enquiries and orders to: University Microfilms Inc.
300 North Zeeb Road, P.O. Box 1346
Ann Arbor, MI 48106-1346 (USA)

Subscription orders: Orders can be placed at agencies, bookstores, directly with the
Publisher S. Karger AG, P.O. Box,
CH–4009 Basel (Switzerland)
or with any of the following distributors:
Deutschland: S. Karger GmbH, Postfach
D–79095 Freiburg
France: Librairie Luginbühl
36, bd de Latour-Maubourg
F–75007 Paris
Great Britain, Ireland: S. Karger Publishers
58 Grove Hill Road
Tunbridge Wells, Kent TN1 1SP, UK
USA: S. Karger Publishers, Inc.
26 West Avon Road, P.O. Box 529
Farmington, CT 06085, USA
India, Bangladesh, Sri Lanka:
Panther Publishers Private Ltd.
39, 6th Cross
Wilson Gardens
Bangalore 560 027, India
Japan: Katakura Libri, Inc.
2F, Marushima Bldg, 4-6-17, Yushima,
Bunkyo-ku, Tokyo 113-0034, Japan

Change of address: Both old and new address should be sent to the subscription source.

Single issues and back volumes: Information can be obtained through the Publisher.

Advertising: Correspondence and rate requests should be addressed to the Publisher.

Bibliographic indices: This journal is regularly listed in bibliographic services, including *Current Contents®*.

Hæmostasis

List of Editors

KARGER

Fax + 41 61 306 12 34
E-Mail karger@karger.ch
www.karger.com

The Journal Home Page is available at:
www.karger.com/journals/hae

List of Editors (continued)

KARGER

Fax+ 41 61 306 12 34
E-Mail karger@karger.ch
www.karger.com

The Journal Home Page is available at:
www.karger.com/journals/hae

Hæmostasis

Thrombosis and Haemostasis Issues in Cancer

International Conference, Bergamo
November 2–4, 2001

Lectures and Abstracts

Editors
Anna Falanga, Bergamo, Italy
Benjamin Brenner, Haifa, Israel
Frederick R. Rickles, Washington, D.C., USA

8 figures and 7 tables, 2001

KARGER
Basel · Freiburg · Paris · London · New York · New Delhi · Bangkok · Singapore · Tokyo · Sydney

S. Karger
Medical and Scientific Publishers
Basel · Freiburg · Paris · London
New York · New Delhi · Bangkok
Singapore · Tokyo · Sydney

Drug Dosage
The authors and the publisher have exerted every effort to ensure that drug selection and dosage set forth in this text are in accord with current recommendations and practice at the time of publication. However, in view of ongoing research, changes in government regulations, and the constant flow of information relating to drug therapy and drug reactions, the reader is urged to check the package insert for each drug for any change in indications and dosage and for added warnings and precautions. This is particularly important when the recommended agent is a new and/or infrequently employed drug.

Printed in Italy by CPZ Litografia sas,
Costa di Mezzate
ISBN 3–8055–7337–5

KARGER

Fax+41 61 306 12 34
E-Mail karger@karger.ch
www.karger.com

Hæmostasis

Vol. 31, Suppl. 1, 2001

Contents

KARGER

Fax +41 61 306 12 34
E-Mail karger@karger.ch
www.karger.com

Access to full text and tables of contents,
including tentative ones for forthcoming issues:
www.karger.com/journals/hae/hae_bk.htm

Hæmostasis

Vol. 31, Suppl. 1, 2001

Preface

This volume contains the proceedings of the 'International Conference on Thrombosis and Hemostasis Issues in Cancer', held at the Congress Center Giovanni XXIII, in Bergamo, Italy from 2 to 4 November, 2001.
This conference is designed to focus on hemostatic system derangements occurring in malignancy, which lead to thrombosis and hemorrhagic syndromes in these patients. Thrombosis is a well-recognized complication of cancer and can contribute significantly to the morbidity and mortality of this disease. Coagulation/bleeding syndromes are rare, but life-threathening, and typically occur in acute leukemias.
Numerous pathogenetic mechanisms have been identified showing that malignant cells can interact with and influence all of the components of the hemostatic system, including blood cells, (i.e. platelets, leukocytes and endothelial cells).

The aim of the conference is to review recent advances in the pathogenesis, prevention and treatment of thrombohemorrhagic complications in cancer patients. We are bringing together leading researchers and clinicians and providing an environment where active exchange of important information and topics of research can take place. On the basis of our current understanding of the molecular mechanisms of pathological thrombus formation in cancer, new approaches to antithrombotic therapy have been attempted, and some of them have proved to be successful. In this congress, various aspects of antithrombotic therapy are discussed with regard to efficacy, safety and issues of cost effectiveness.

The conference is divided into different sessions covering the following issues:
a) pathogenetic mechanisms, showing the plausibility of the association of clotting with malignancy; b) the link between tumor induced angiogenesis and thrombosis; c) clinical syndromes associated with malignancy (from subclinical hypercoagulable conditions to systemic syndromes, such as disseminated intravascular coagulation and thrombotic microangiopathies); and finally d) new concepts of prophylaxis and treatment of these complications in patients with malignancy.

We sincerely hope that this volume will enhance the overall knowledge on the interactions between the hemostatic system and malignant disease and will provide useful information to the readers on the prevention and management of thrombotic complications in cancer patients by serving as a reference and a source of inspiration.

We wish to thank all participants for their contributions.

Anna Falanga
Benjamin Brenner
Frederick R Rickles

KARGER

Fax +41 61 306 12 34
E-Mail karger@karger.ch
www.karger.com

Accessible online at:
www.karger.com/journals/hae

Hæmostasis
Vol. 31, Suppl. 1, 2001

Lectures

Haemostasis

Lecture Index

Haemostasis 2001;31(suppl. 1)

Tumor cells and hemostasis

Angiogenesis

Epidemiological aspects of thrombosis in cancer

Systemic Syndromes

Platelets, fibrinolysis and cancer

Prevention and treatment of VTE in cancer

Hæmostasis

Lectures

Haemostasis 2001;31(suppl. 1):1-4

Tumor cells and hemostasis

Tumor cell prothrombotic properties

ANNA FALANGA
Division of Hematology, Dept. Hematology-Oncology, Ospedali Riuniti, Bergamo - Italy.

Abstract
Thrombin generation and fibrin formation are constantly determined in patients with malignancy, who are at increased risk of thromboembolic complications. Most importantly, fibrin formation is also involved in the processes of tumor spread and metastasis.
Activation of blood coagulation in cancer is a complex phenomenon, involving many different pathways of the hemostatic system and numerous interactions of the tumor cell with other blood cells, including platelet, monocyte and endothelial cell. Tumor cells possess the capacity to interact with all parts of the hemostatic system. They can directly activate the coagulation cascade by producing their own procoagulant factors or they can stimulate the prothrombotic properties of other blood cell components. All of the mechanisms are not entirely understood, however research studies in the last ten years have greatly improved our knowledge of tumor-promoted pro-thrombotic functions.

Introduction

Malignancy is a recognized acquired thrombophilic condition. Patients with cancer are at significantly increased risk of thrombosis, particularly after surgery or other predisposing conditions (chemotherapy, radiotherapy, long term bedrest, trauma) [1]. It is also well known that idiopathic venous thromboembolism can represent the earliest clinical manifestation of cancer [2], and a 'hypercoagulable state' is present in the majority of cancer patients, even without clinical symptoms of thrombosis. Abnormalities in laboratory coagulation tests show varying degrees of blood clotting activation in these patients [3], demonstrating that a process of fibrin formation and removal is continuously ongoing during the development of malignancy. Notably, fibrin formation plays a role not only in thrombogenesis but also in tumor progression [4], as will be extensively discussed by various scientists in this Conference.
Histological studies of tumor specimens have documented the presence of fibrin or platelet plugs in and around many types of tumors, suggesting that activation of blood coagulation can occur locally at the tumor level [5]. Indeed tumor cells possess the full capacity to activate all the components of the hemostatic system, although general mechanisms related to the host response to the tumor (i.e., the acute-phase reaction, paraprotein production, inflammation, necrosis, hemodynamic disorders) can also contribute to clotting activation in malignancy. However, a prominent role is attributed to tumor-specific clot promoting mechanisms.

Tumor cell prothrombotic mechanisms

Malignant cells can interact with the hemostatic system in multiple ways.
The principal prothrombotic properties of tumor cells are:
1) the capacity to produce and release procoagulant activities, fibrinolytic proteins, and inflammatory cytokines, i.e. interleukin-1ß (IL-1ß), tumour necrosis factor (TNF-α) and vascular endothelial growth factor (VEGF); and,

KARGER
Fax +41 61 306 12 34
E-Mail karger@karger.ch
www.karger.com

0301-0147/00/0309/0001$17.50/0

Accessible online at:
www.karger.com/journals/hae

Anna Falanga
Dipartimento di Ematologia-Oncologia
Azienda Ospedaliera Ospedali Riuniti
Largo Barozzi, 1 24128 BERGAMO
Tel. +39/035/269491 Fax +39/035/266147
annafalanga@yahoo.com

2) the capacity to interact with host cells, including endothelial cells lining the blood vessels, monocytes, platelets and neutrophils.

1. Tumor procoagulants, fibrinolytic proteins, and cytokines:

Procoagulant activities (PCA)

These properties enable tumor cells to promote fibrin formation at the site of tumor microenviroment. Tumor cells may express different types of procoagulants, the best characterized of which are: Tissue Factor and Cancer Procoagulant.

Tissue factor (TF) is a 47 kDa transmembrane glycoprotein which forms a complex with factor VII (FVII)/FVIIa: the TF/FVII complex triggers blood coagulation by proteolytically activating factors IX and X [6]. TF is the cellular procoagulant found in normal cells, including endothelial cells and monocyte-macrophages. However, these cells do not express TF in normal resting conditions, but expose this procoagulant in response to pro-inflammatory stimuli, i.e. the cytokines IL-1β and TNFα and bacterial endotoxins [7]. Differently from normal cells, malignant cells constitutively express TF. In addition to activating blood coagulation, TF has the capacity of regulating VEGF expression in tumor cells and in vascular endothelium [4], which represents an important pro-angiogenetic mechanism.

Cancer Procoagulant (CP) is a 68 kDa cysteine proteinase (EC 3.4.22.26) with 674 amino acid residues and no detectable carbohydrates [8]. It activates factor X independently of FVII and cleaves the factor X heavy chain at a different site compared to other known factor X activators. CP has been found in extracts of malignant cells or in amnion-chorion tissues but not in extracts of normally differentiated cells [9]. CP antigen has been identified in the sera of cancer patients and found to be elevated in 85% of the study subjects.

TF and CP have been identified in several human and animal tumor tissues. The two proteins are different in nature; therefore, different methods for processing the tissue sample are required to meet the optimal assay conditions to quantify each of these procoagulants [10].

We have particularly focused on the PCA of leukemic cells. Recent data show that differentiating treatment with all-trans-Retinoic Acid (ATRA) of acute promyelocytic leukemia (APL) cells down-regulates the expression of CP and TF both 'in vitro' and 'in vivo'. The demonstration that this effect parallels the improvement of the plasma hypercoagulation parameters in patients with APL provides the first evidence 'in vivo' for a role of tumor cell PCA in the hemostatic complications associated with malignancy [11]. Further, CP activity is modulated by ATRA only in differentiating, whereas TF activity is significantly reduced in all cell lines, regardless of their differentiation status. These results are in agreement with the characteristics of the two procoagulants and provide support for the concept that CP is a differentiation-dependent protein.

Fibrinolytic activities

Tumor cells can express all the proteins regulating the fibrinolytic system, including the urokinase-type plasminogen activator (u-PA), the tissue-type plasminogen activator (t-PA), and the fibrinolysis inhibitors PAI-1 and PAI-2 [10]. Among the activators, u-PA is the most widely expressed within malignant lesions. Furthermore, cancer cells can carry the specific plasminogen activator receptor (uPAR) on their membranes. The presence of these receptors favors the assembly of all the fibrinolytic components on tumor cell membranes, facilitating the activation of the fibrinolytic cascade. The finding of impaired plasma fibrinolytic activity in patients with solid tumors represents another tumor-associated prothrombotic mechanism [10]. Importantly, fibrinolysis proteins can play a role in tumor cell proliferation, invasion and metastasis.

Cytokines

Tumor cells produce inflammatory cytokines, including TNF-α, IL-1ß and VEGF. Tumour cell-derived TNF-α and IL-1ß can induce the expression of TF procoagulant activity by endothelial cells. They also down-regulate the expression of endothelial cell thrombomodulin (TM), the surface high-affinity receptor for thrombin. The TM-thrombin complex activates the protein C system, which in turn functions as a potent anticoagulant. TF up-regulation and TM down-regulation lead to a prothrombotic condition of the vascular wall [3, 10]. The same cytokines stimulate endothelial cells to produce the fibrinolysis inhibitor PAI-1. Inhibition of fibrinolysis further contributes to the prothrombotic potential of endothelial cells. In addition, the production of VEGF by malignant cells may significantly affect the functions of microvascular vessels in proximity of the tumor and may play an important role in tumor neo-angiogenesis [4]. Further, VEGF is chemotactic for macrophages and can induce TF procoagulant activity of monocyte and endothelial cell. Interestingly, the expression of TF by tumor cells upregulates the transcription of VEGF in these cells. Finally, TF modulates the expression of VEGF by endothelial cells, a function that can have important implications in tumor neo-vascularization [4]. Regulation of VEGF synthesis by TF in malignant cells and vascular cells provides an important link in cancer patients between activation of coagulation, inflammation, thrombosis and tumor progression and metastasis.

2. Tumor cell-Host cell interactions

Studies of laboratory parameters demonstrate the activation/perturbation of several cellular systems 'in vivo' in cancer patients. Indeed, findings of elevated levels of plasma endothelial markers (e.g. von Willebrand factor, thrombomodulin, soluble E-selectin, tissue-type plasminogen activator [t-PA] and PAI-1) indicate the activation of hemostasis at the endothelium site, especially during chemotherapy [3, 10]. Further, the increase in tissue factor procoagulant activity (PCA) expressed by circulating mononuclear cells shows that this cellular compartment has become activated [7]. Finally, the detection of high levels of platelet membrane specific glycoproteins (e.g. CD62 and CD63), which are exposed upon activation, provides evidence for platelet activation 'in vivo' in malignant conditions [3]. Recently, neutrophil activation in patients with myeloproliferative disorders has also been demonstrated [12].

Tumour cells can interact with the endothelium essentially by their capacity to synthesize and release inflammatory cytokines, as above described. These cells can also directly adhere to endothelial cells and to the extracellular matrix through membrane adhesion molecules. Endothelial cells activated by IL-1ß or TNF-α increase the exposure on their membranes of counter-receptors for the tumor adhesion molecules. The malignant cells attached to the vessel wall may play a key role in promoting localized clotting activation and thrombus formation by releasing their cytokine content and favoring the adhesion and arrest of other cells, including leukocytes and platelets. The adhesion of tumor cells to leukocytes or to vascular cells may also facilitate cell migration and extravasation. In addition, the TF-induced expression of VEGF by endothelial cells may have implications in tumor neovascularization.

Platelets can be activated by cells from human and experimental tumors. Upon activation they aggregate and release their granule contents, as shown by 'in vitro' and 'in vivo' studies. Tumor cells, or membrane vesicles spontaneously shed from tumour cells in the medium, can directly aggregate platelets 'in vitro'. Alternatively, they can induce platelet aggregation through the release of proaggregatory mediators including ADP, thrombin and a cathepsin-like cysteine proteinase [10].

Tumor cells interact with monocyte-macrophages. These cells circulate in the blood stream, or are localized on the vascular wall in response to inflammatory stimuli. They are also part of the lymphoreticular infiltrate of the tumor mass. Similarly to endothelial cells, mononuclear phagocytes do not constitutively express TF, but generate this procoagulant on their surface in response to different stimuli, including bacterial endotoxin, inflammatory particles, complement proteins, immune complexes and lymphokines. 'In vitro' studies show that tumor cells and/or tumor cell products can induce the expression of monocyte TF [7]. Mononuclear cell activation may occur 'in vivo' as well. Indeed, tumor-associated macrophages harvested from experimental and human tumors express significantly more TF than control cells, contributing to localized fibrin deposition within tumor tissues. Further, circulating monocytes from patient with different types of cancer have been shown to express increased TF activity [7, 10], thus contributing to the activation of the patient hemostatic system.

References

1. Rickles FR, Levine MN. Epidemiology of thrombosis in cancer. Acta Haematologica 2001; 106: 6-12.
2. Prandoni P, Lensing AWA, Buller HR et al. Deep-vein thrombosis and the incidence of subsequent symptomatic cancer. New Engl J Med 1992; 327: 1128-33.
3. Falanga A. Mechanisms of hypercoagulation in malignancy and during chemotherapy. Haemostasis 1998: 28 (suppl 3): 50-60.
4. Rickles FR, Falanga A. Molecular basis for the relationship between thrombosis and cancer. Thromb Res 2001; 102 (Suppl.): V215-V224.
5. Donati MB, Falanga A. Pathogenetic mechanisms of thrombosis in malignancy. Acta Haematologica 2001; 106: 18-24.
6. Nemerson Y.: The tissue factor pathway of blood coagulation. Sem Hematol 1992; 29: 170-6.
7. Semeraro N, Colucci M. Tissue factor in health and disease. Thromb Haemost 1997; 78: 759-64.
8. Falanga A, Gordon SG.: Isolation and characterization of cancer procoagulant: A Cysteine proteinase from malignant tissue. Biochemistry 1985; 24: 5558-5567.
9. Gale AJ, Gordon SG. Update on tumor cell procoagulant factors. Acta Haematologica 2001; 106: 25-32.
10. Falanga A, Rickels FR. Pathophisiology of the thrombophilic state in the cancer patients. Sem Thromb Haemost 1999; 25: 173-82.
11. Barbui T, Finazzi G, & Falanga A. The impact of all-trans-retinoic acid on the coagulopathy of acute promyelocytic leukemia. Blood 1998; 91: 3093-3102.
12. Falanga A, Marchetti M, Evangelista V et al. Polymorphonuclear leukocyte activation and hemostasis in patients with Essential Thrombocythemia and Polycythemia Vera. Blood 2000; 96: 4261-6.

Hæmostasis

Lectures

Haemostasis 2001;31(suppl. 1):5-7

Molecular regulation of blood clotting in tumor biology

WOLFRAM RUF
Department of Immunology and Vascular Biology, The Scripps Research Institute; La Jolla, CA, U.S.A

Abstract
TF expression is a hallmark of cancer progression. The procoagulant functions of TF that lead to thrombin generation are critically important to support metastasis, in part through the generation of fibrin that assures prolonged arrest of tumor cells in target organs. In addition, the coagulation initiation complex, i.e. TF-VIIa-Xa, generates autocrine cell signaling though protease activated receptors. A cooperation of the TF cytoplasmic domain with protease signaling may explain the diverse contributions of TF to metastasis and angiogenesis.

Introduction
Tissue factor is the principal cellular activator of the coagulation cascade. TF expression in cancer is frequent. Large scale genomic analysis of cancer identified TF as part of a gene cluster that is upregulated in the course of dedifferentiation to a "mesynchymal" phenotype [1], linking TF to cancer progression. Activation of coagulation requires the contact of a TF expressing cell with the blood or plasma. In cancer biology this can occur either during tumor angiogenesis, when the hyperpermeable tumor vasculature allows for extravasation of plasma components, or during metastatic tumor dissemination, when tumor cells travel in the blood stream. As a consequence, signs of activation of the coagulation cascade, i.e. clinical thrombosis and prominent tumor associated fibrin deposition, have early on been recognized as a hallmark of malignancy.

Biochemistry of TF initiated coagulation
How TF functions in the initiation of coagulation have been defined in detail by biochemical and crystallographic methods [2]. TF forms a stoichiometric complex with either factor VII or the active enzyme VIIa. VIIa has the unique property to be essentially inactive in the absence of TF and, as a consequence, VIIa is circulating with considerable half-life in the blood. Binding of VIIa to cell surface expressed TF results in allosteric activation of the labile enzyme, thus triggering the initiating events of blood clotting. TF not only serves as the activator of VIIa, but has more important functions in orchestrating the recognition of macromolecular substrates, i.e. factors IX and X. The current model suggests that the Gla-domain of substrate X makes interactions with both, cofactor TF and enzyme VIIa, and that the protease domains of substrate and enzyme are in contact. The TF initiation complex is thus a ternary unit consisting of TF-VIIa-X. The extended interactions provide all the required binding energy for X to specifically interact with TF-VIIa, and the cleavage of the scissile bond of X appears to occur secondary to ternary complex formation. Because of the multiple interactions in the ternary complex, product Xa has measurable affinity for TF-VIIa and a transient ternary TF-VIIa-Xa complex is predicted to exist.
Notably, the physiological inhibitor of the TF pathway, TFPI, preferably recognizes this ternary TF-VIIa-Xa complex by simultaneously binding the first and second Kunitz inhibitory domains to VIIa and Xa, respectively.
Moreover, a nematode-derived inhibitor, NAPc2, that is under investigation as a TF-specific antithrombotic, can similarly lock in the TF-VIIa-Xa complex. However, NAPc2, unlike TFPI, binds Xa outside of the catalytic center and is capable to interact with substrate X to provide a substrate-delivered inhibitory mechanism of TF-VIIa. The biochemical studies of the cell surface initiation reaction thus established unique functional characteristics that differ significantly from rules for proteases, such as thrombin, that primarily act as solution phase enzymes.

KARGER
Fax +41 61 306 12 34
E-Mail karger@karger.ch
www.karger.com

0301-0147/00/0309/0001$17.50/0

Accessible online at:
www.karger.com/journals/hae

Wolfram Ruf
The Scripps Research Institute - Department of Immunology, C204
10550 North Torrey Pines Road
La Jolla CA 92037 - USA
Tel. +1/858/7842748 - Fax +1/858/7848480
ruf@scripps.edu

Coupling of initiation of coagulation to protease activated receptor signaling

The functional characteristics of the TF initiation complex have proven to be crucial for the understanding of cell signaling events that are triggered by the coagulation reaction. Thrombin has long been appreciated as a signaling protease in its hemostatic function to activate platelets through activation of protease activated receptors, i.e. PAR1, PAR3, and PAR4 [3]. Thrombin recognizes and cleaves a substrate-like sequence in the extracellular domain of these receptors. The cleavage exposes a new amino-terminus that serves as a tethered ligand to interact with the binding pocket of the receptor to trigger the G-protein coupled signaling events. Although originally identified as "thrombin-receptors", PARs represent more generalized sensors of extracellular proteolytic activity. In particular, PAR2, which is not cleaved by thrombin, can be activated by several proteases, including Xa and TF-VIIa. Xa and plasmin also activate the prototypical thrombin receptor PAR1, albeit with lower efficiency. The slower receptor cleavage does not necessarily result in decreased biological responses, such as induction of angiogenesis promoting genes [4]. However, there have been concerns whether the upstream proteases Xa and TF-VIIa can promote significant cell signaling under in vivo conditions where thrombin, a much more efficient signaling protease, is simultaneously generated. We found that TF-VIIa dependent X activation on cells produced Xa-dependent cell signaling that was not expected from the low concentration of Xa that was detected under the experimental conditions [5]. Moreover, equivalent amounts of Xa generated by the intrinsic VIIIa-IXa complex did not result in cell signaling through PAR1 or PAR2. These data suggested that Xa in the ternary TF-VIIa-Xa complex may be signaling competent. In support of this concept, PAR1 and PAR2 activation was highly efficient in the presence of the nematode inhibitor NAPc2 which traps the ternary TF-VIIa-Xa complex. The initiation reaction thus generates a transient TF-VIIa-Xa signaling complex that triggers cells in an autocrine manner. TFPI may subsequently "lock in" this complex and inhibit its function. Thus, the signaling event may occur in the absence of massive activation of the coagulation cascade that requires the release of product Xa.

Fig. 1: Schematic representation of the functional roles of TF in tumor cell metastasis.

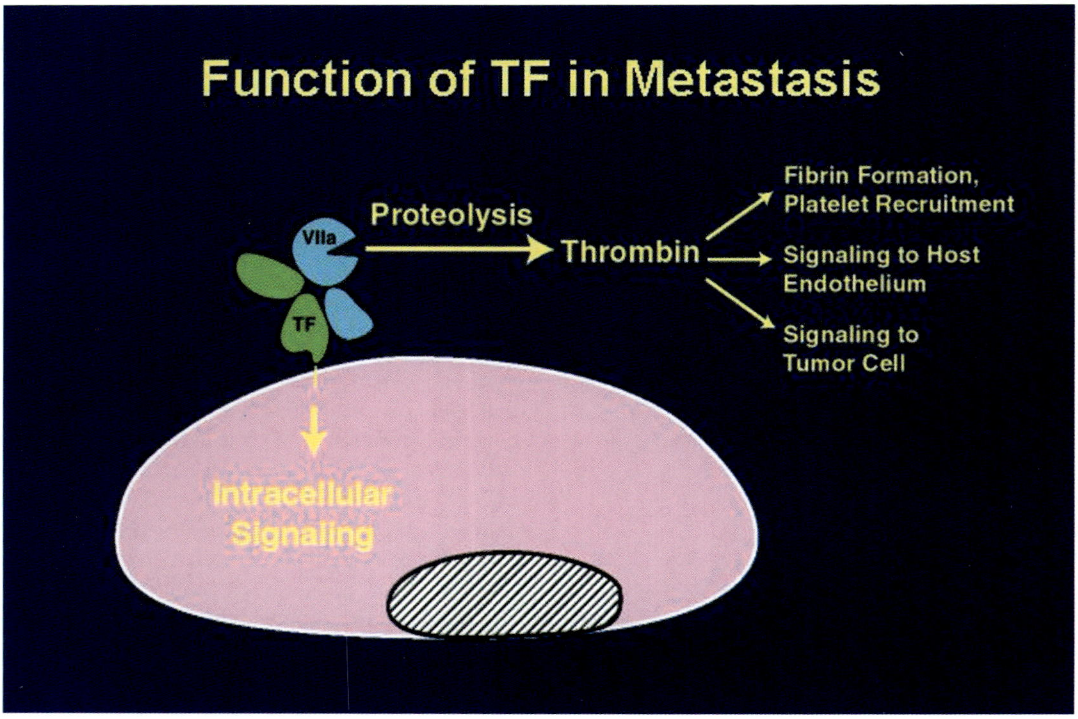

TF-dependent metastasis

Cell signaling events have been appreciated as of importance for TF-dependent tumor cell metastasis. Aggressive melanoma cells isolated from patients typically express TF and show TF-dependent experimental metastasis in immuno-deficient animals [6]. The prometastatic functions of TF can also be recapitulated in Chinese hamster ovary cells which allowed us to define the domains in TF that contribute to the metastatic process [7]. These studies demonstrated that both the TF cytoplasmic domain and the VIIa-binding extracellular domain make equally important contributions to the prometastatic functions of TF (Fig. 1). In all experimental models, thrombin was found to be a central player, reflecting the requirement for fibrin formation that may stabilize implantation and/or platelet recruitment. Additional roles for thrombin have not been conclusively established. Signaling to the PAR1 expressing endothelium may facilitate adhesion. All metastatic tumor cells express PAR1 and autocrine cell signaling may play an additional important role in the metastatic process. The essential contributions of the TF cytoplasmic domain and its phosphorylation motifs in the metastatic process suggest that TF may directly participate in these autocrine cell signaling events. Whether the cytoplasmic domain acts independently or in the context of PAR signaling event remains an exciting area of investigation.

References

1. Ross D, Scherf U, Eisen M, et al. Systematic variation in gene expression patterns in human cancer cell lines. Nature Genet 2000; 24:227-235.
2. Ruf W and Dickinson CD Allosteric regulation of the cofactor-dependent serine protease coagulation factor VIIa. Trends Cardiovasc Med 1998; 8:350-356.
3. Coughlin SR Thrombin signalling and protease-activated receptors. Nature 2000; 407:258-264.
4. Riewald M, Kravchenko VV, Petrovan RJ, et al. Gene induction by coagulation factor Xa is mediated by activation of PAR-1. Blood 2001; 97:3109-3116.
5. Riewald, M, Ruf, W Mechanistic coupling of protease signaling and initiation of coagulation by tissue factor. Proc Natl Acad Sci USA 2001; 98:7742-7747.
6. Mueller BM, Reisfeld RA, Edgington TS, et al. Expression of tissue factor by melanoma cells promotes efficient hematogenous metastasis. Proc Natl Acad Sci USA 1992; 89:11832-11836.
7. Mueller BM and Ruf W. Requirement for binding of catalytically active factor VIIa in tissue factor dependent experimental metastasis. J Clin Invest 1998; 101:1372-1378.

Hæmostasis

Lectures

Haemostasis 2001;31(suppl. 1):8-10

Biochemistry of cancer procoagulant

WOJCIECH P MIELICKI
Department of Pharmaceutical Biochemistry, Medical University of Lodz, Lodz, Poland

Abstract
Cancer procoagulant (CP), EC3.4.22.26, is a cysteine proteinase produced by malignant or fetal tissue. It is a single chain Mr 68 kDa protein containing no carbohydrates. Prevalent amino acids are Ser (19.15), Gly (18.7%), Glu (12.5%), Lys (8.1%) and Asp (7.1%). Amino-acid sequence of CP is not determined yet. The natural substrates for CP are coagulation factor X and probably PAR-1 receptor. However, the peptidyl bond in factor X molecule hydrolyzed by CP is different from the bond recognized by other known FX-activators. Peptidyl chromogenic substrates hydrolyzed by CP are those with Pro at P2 and Arg or Lys at P1 position. Factor X-activating activity of CP is inhibited by number of various inhibitors: peptidyl diazomethyl ketones, iodoacetamide, mercuric chloride, PMSF, leupeptin and antipain. It has been demonstrated that E-64, a specific inhibitor of cysteine proteinases, inhibits CP reversible acting as a competitive inhibitor of the enzyme. The CP activity is modulated by the presence of divalent metal ions in the reaction environment. Ca^{2+}, Cd^{2+}, Mg^{2+} and Mn^{2+} ions potentiate the procoagulant activity when Cu^{2+}, Fe^{2+}, Sn^{2+} and Zn^{2+} ions inactivate CP.

Introduction
Studies on factors potentially responsible for activation of the blood clotting cascade in malignant disease led to the discovery of a unique proteolytic activator of coagulation factor X (Gordon et al., 1975). Since the protein, able to promote blood clotting in vitro, has been obtained from malignant tissue (rabbit V2 carcinoma) it has been named Cancer Procoagulant (CP). Later CP-like activity has been found in extracts from many experimental and human solid tumors and leukemic cells but not in normally differentiated tissues (Gordon and Mielicki, 1997). It seems that the only one non-malignant tissue containing CP is fetal tissue and amnion-chorion membranes (Falanga and Gordon, 1985a). During past two decades many of structural and biochemical properties of CP have been described. However, there is still no information concerning the CP amino-acid sequence as well as nothing is known on the gene encoding CP. This presentation intends to briefly summarize the available data describing biochemical properties of cancer procoagulant.

Structural data
According to the studies performed over 15 years ago cancer procoagulant isolated from rabbit V2 carcinoma is a single chain protein of molecular weight about 68 kDa, pI=4.8, containing no carbohydrate component. Prevalent amino-acids in the CP molecule are: Ser (19.1%), Gly (18.7%), Glu (12.5%), Lys (8.1%) and Asp (7.1%) (Falanga and Gordon, 1985b). There is indirect evidence that CP moiety contains γ-carboxyglutamic acid (Gla) residues (Roncaglioni et al., 1989), however, the direct analysis of Gla content in CP has not been performed yet. There is direct evidence that CP contains at least two different metal-binding sites: one for calcium and magnesium, the second for manganese and cadmium. The divalent metals are responsible for correct conformation of the molecule (Mielicki et al., 1994a, Mielicki and Sobolewska, 2001).

Enzymatic properties
Cancer procoagulant activates plasma blood clotting cascade by a proteolytic cleavage of the heavy chain of coagulation factor X. However, the site of FX hydrolysis by CP is slightly different from the site cleaved by FIXa/FVIIIa, FVIIa/TF or procoagulant from Russell's viper venom (RVV). CP recognizes the peptidyl bond between Tyr^{21} and Asp^{22} while the other procoagulants activate FX at Arg^{52} (Gordon and Mourad, 1991). For a long time factor X was considered as the only known physiologic substrate for CP. Recent experiments on stimulation of blood platelet adhesion by CP suggest another possible protein substrate for the enzyme. Although the cellular activation events by CP may be initiated by a standard receptor (ligand-binding interactions), it seems that CP competes with thrombin for the same

KARGER
Fax +41 61 306 12 34
E-Mail karger@karger.ch
www.karger.com

0301-0147/00/0309/0001$17.50/0

Accessible online at:
www.karger.com/journals/hae

Wojciech P. Mielicki
Department of Pharmaceutical Biochemistry - Medical University of Lodz
Ul Muszynskiego 1 - Lodz 90151 - POLAND
Tel. +48/42/6785524 - Fax +48/42/6788398
wojtek77@friko2.onet.pl - mielicki@friko2.onet.pl

receptor on the blood platelet surface, called protease-activated receptor 1 (PAR-1) (Olas et al., 2000).

Valuable tools for studying of the active site of proteinases are synthetic, peptidyl chromogenic (or fluorogenic) substrates. Many various peptidyl sequences have been analyzed as potential substrates for CP. It has been demonstrated that CP cleaves the substrates containing Pro or Pip at P2 and Arg or Lys at P1 position, however, the maximum velocity of the reaction was very low. The best synthetic substrates hydrolyzed by CP are: H-D-Ile-Pro-Arg-pNA, N-p-Tos-Gly-Pro-Arg-pNA, H-D-Ala-Pro-Arg-pNA, N-p-Tos-Gly-Pro-Lys-pNA and pyroGlu-Pro-Arg-pNA. Surprisingly, CP does not cleave the sequence: x-Lys-Pro^{P2}-Tyr^{P1}-, the one recognized by the enzyme in FX (Mielicki et al., 1997). This suggests that active site recognition of CP on native, high molecular weight protein substrates may be directed by secondary or tertiary protein configuration rather then primary sequence alone, or/and by primary sequence also on the carboxyl side (P') of the cleaved bond. There also may be the protein-protein interactions outside the active site of CP necessary for the correct fitting of the substrate in the active site.

Inhibitors and activators of CP

Various types of natural and synthetic proteinase inhibitors and metal ions inhibit the enzymatic activity of cancer procoagulant. The effectiveness of most of the inhibitors increases in the presence of reducing agent in the reaction environment. However, it has been found that mercuric chloride blocks the CP activity better without the reducing compounds. It has been demonstrated that following non-specific cysteine proteinase inhibitors inhibit the CP activity: iodoacetamide, p-chloromercuric benzoate, leupeptin, antipain and PMSF (Moore 1992, Mielicki et al. 1994b). Moreover, cancer procoagulant activity is inhibited by peptidyl diazomethyl ketones, considered as specific cysteine proteinase inhibitors (Falanga et al. 1989). Also it was determined that specific cysteine proteinase inhibitor E-64 (trans-epoxysuccinyl-L-leucylamido-(4-guanidino)butane) inhibits CP activity, acting as reversible, competitive inhibitor of the procoagulant. The inhibition constant Ki calculated for the reaction was 0.128 mM (Mielicki and Sobolewska, 2001). CP activity is not inhibited by natural protease inhibitors: α2-macroglobulin, α1-antiprotease, antithrombin III/heparin, cystatin, cystamine and α1-antichymotrypsin. Inhibition of the CP factor X-activating activity by specific cysteine proteinase inhibitors allowed for the classification of the enzyme as a cysteine proteinase (EC 3.4.22.26).

Cancer procoagulant seems to be an enzyme regulated allosterically. Certain divalent metal ions may modulate the factor X-activating activity of CP. It has been proved that the metals do not participate directly in the reaction within the active site, but metal-protein interaction takes place in other region of the enzyme. Most likely the divalent metals are responsible for active, or inactive conformation of CP. Preincubation of CP with 1 mM chlorides of copper, iron, tin or zinc almost completely block the activity. On the other hand, the other divalent ions are required for the activity of CP. It has been demonstrated that 7 mM calcium or magnesium chloride, 0.1 mM manganese chloride or 1 mM cadmium chloride were necessary to obtain an active CP able to hydrolysis of FX (Mielicki et al. 1994a, Mielicki and Sobolewska 2001).

References

1. Falanga A and Gordon SG. Comparison of properties of cancer procoagulant and human amnion-chorion procoagulant. Biochim Biophys Acta 1985a; 831, 161-165.
2. Falanga A and Gordon SG. Isolation and characterization of cancer procoagulant: a cysteine proteinase from malignant tissue. Biochemistry 1985b; 24, 5558-5567.
3. Falanga A, Shaw E, Donati MB, Consonni R, Barbui T, Gordon SG. Inhibition of cancer procoagulant by peptidyl diazomethyl ketones and peptidyl sulfonium salts. Thromb Res 1989; 54, 389-398.
4. Gordon SG, Franks JJ, Lewis B. Cancer procoagulant: a factor X-activating procoagulant from malignant tissue. Thromb Res 1975; 6, 127-137.
5. Gordon SG and Mourad AM. The site of activation of factor X by cancer procoagulant. Blood Coag Fibrinol 1991; 2, 735-739.
6. Gordon SG and Mielicki WP. Cancer procoagulant: a factor X-activator, tumor marker and growth factor from malignant tissue. Blood Coag Fibrinol 1997; 8, 73-86.
7. Mielicki WP, Kozwich DL, Kramer LC, Gordon SG. Effect of divalent ions on the activity of cancer procoagulant. Arch Biochem Biophys 1994a; 314, 165-170.
8. Mielicki WP, Tagawa M, Gordon SG. New immunocapture enzyme (ICE) assay for quantification of cancer procoagulant activity: studies of inhibitors. Thromb Haemost 1994b; 71, 456-460.
9. Mielicki WP, Mielicka E, Gordon SG. Cancer procoagulant activity studies using synthetic chromogenic substrates. Thromb Res 1997; 87, 251-256.
10. Mielicki WP and Sobolewska M. Cancer procoagulant (EC 3.4.22.26): the kinetics of its inhibition by E-64 and modulation of the activity by cadmium, copper and tin ions. Cancer Res Therapy Ctrl 2001; 11, 135-141.
11. Moore WR. The purification and properties of cancer procoagulant from murine tumors. Biochem Biophys Res Commun 1992; 184, 819-824.
12. Olas B, Wachowicz B, Mielicki WP, Buczynski A. Free radicals are involved in cancer procoagulant –induced platelet activation. Thromb Res 2000; 97, 169-175.
13. Roncaglioni MC, Falanga A, Bolognese Dalessandro AP, Alessio MG, Casali B, Donati MB. Evidence of warfarin-sensitive cancer procoagulant in V2 carcinoma. Haematologica, 1989; 74, 143-147.

Hæmostasis

Lectures

Haemostasis 2001;31(suppl. 1):11-15

Fibrinogen and tumor cell metastasis

JOSEPH S PALUMBO [1], JAY L DEGEN [2]

1 Divisions of Hematology/Oncology and
2 Developmental Biology, Children's Hospital Research Foundation
and University of Cincinnati College of Medicine.

Abstract

Detailed studies of tumor cell-associated procoagulants and fibrinolytic factors have strongly suggested that local thrombin and plasmin generation may be important in tumor progression. Given that one target for both these serine proteases is fibrinogen, a logical extension of this hypothesis is that local fibrin deposition and dissolution may be key determinants of tumor growth and/or dissemination. To directly test this concept, we initiated studies of tumor growth, experimental metastasis, and spontaneous metastasis in C57Bl/6-inbred mice with and without fibrinogen. Using two established C57Bl/6-derived tumor cell lines, Lewis lung carcinoma and B16-BL6 melanoma, fibrinogen deficiency was found to strongly diminish, but not prevent, the development of lung metastases in both experimental and spontaneous metastasis assays. This difference was not a consequence of any obvious difference in tumor stroma formation or the growth of primary or secondary tumors. Rather, tumor cell fate studies argued that there is an important role of fibrin(ogen) in the sustained adhesion and/or survival of tumor cell emboli within the lung. The specific thrombin inhibitor, hirudin, was also shown to strongly diminish metastatic potential, consistent with earlier reports. More importantly, hirudin was found to further diminish the already low metastatic potential of tumor cells in fibrinogen-deficient mice. We conclude that fibrin(ogen) is a critical determinant of metastatic potential, but thrombin appears to contribute to tumor cell dissemination through at least one fibrinogen-independent mechanism. Further, these findings suggest that therapeutic strategies directed at several hemostatic factors might be useful in the suppression of metastatic disease.

Introduction

An important relationship between cancer biology and specific hemostatic system components (e.g., fibrinogen and plasminogen) has been suspected for decades. Based on the ability of provisional fibrin matrices to support adhesion and migration of many types of cells, including capillary endothelial cells, one leading hypothesis has been that fibrin matrices within solid tumors may support the formation of tumor stroma that ultimately serves as a life-support system for rapidly dividing tumor cells [1]. Similarly, tumor-associated plasminogen activation has also been tightly linked to tumor dissemination. Epidemiological studies have shown that high expression of plasminogen activator (PA), PA receptor or PA inhibitor is associated with a poor prognosis in many types of human cancers. Furthermore, the metastatic potential of transplantable tumor models has been reported in multiple studies to be reduced when PA expression or activity is experimentally modified (e.g., antisense RNA, anticatalytic PA antibodies). The recent generation of mice with selected deficits in fibrinogen, plasminogen, plasminogen activators and plasminogen activator inhibitor (PAI-1) has provided a unique opportunity to directly test the hypothesis that these factors are important determinants of tumor growth and metastasis [2-11]. Below we summarize some of the initial findings made with fibrinogen-deficient mice that point to a role of this key hemostatic factor in tumor dissemination.

Results and Discussion

Hematogenous Metastasis in Fibrinogen-deficient Mice. Studies focusing on the experimental metastasis of Lewis lung carcinoma and B16 melanoma in histocompatible fibrinogen-deficient mice have firmly established that fibrinogen is an important determinant of tumor dissemination in vivo ([9] and see Figure 1). The quantitative reduction in metastatic potential in fibrinogen-deficient mice was

KARGER

Fax +41 61 306 12 34
E-Mail karger@karger.ch
www.karger.com

0301-0147/00/0309/0001$17.50/0

Accessible online at:
www.karger.com/journals/hae

Jay L. Degen
Children's Hospital Research Foundation - Children's Hospital Medical Center
IDR-NRB Room 2042 3333 Burnet Avenue
Cincinnati OH 45229-3039 - USA
Tel. +1/513/6364679 - Fax +1/513/6364317
degenjl@chmcc.org

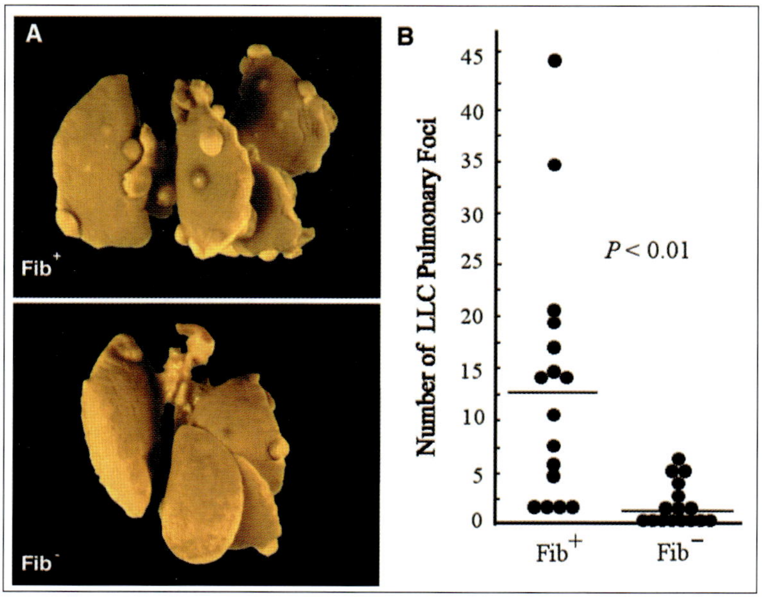

Figure 1

Fibrinogen-deficiency diminishes the metastatic potential of circulating tumor cells.
A) Lungs with representative examples of metastatic pulmonary foci harvested 21 days following intravenous injection of 1 x 10^5 LLC cells into the lateral tail vein of control (top) and fibrinogen-deficient mice (bottom).
B) Scatter plot of the number of surface pulmonary metastases observed in individual mice.
The horizontal bars represent median values for each group. The P value was determined by the Mann Whitney U test.

not the result of any obvious difference in tumor stroma development or tumor growth in metastatic lesions (see below). Rather, tumor cell fate studies point to an important role of fibrin(ogen) in the sustained adhesion and/or survival of tumor cells within the lung. The fact that the specific thrombin inhibitor, hirudin, is also highly effective in diminishing metastatic potential in hematogenous metastasis assays suggests, but does not prove, that tumor cell-mediated conversion of fibrinogen to fibrin may be mechanistically coupled to metastatic success. However, it should be noted that there are multiple targets of thrombin-mediated proteolysis other than fibrinogen that might be relevant to metastatic disease, including factor XI, factor XIII, thrombin-activated fibrinolysis inhibitor (TAFI), protein C, and the G-protein coupled protease-activated receptors-1, -3, and -4. Indeed, the fact that hirudin was found to further diminish the already low metastatic potential of circulating tumor cells in fibrinogen-deficient mice argues that there is at least one target of thrombin-mediated proteolysis other than fibrinogen that is important in metastatic disease. Taken together, the data suggest that fibrinogen is an important determinant of the metastatic potential of circulating tumor cells, but thrombin appears to facilitate tumor dissemination through at least one fibrin(ogen)-independent mechanism. Of course, the precise mechanism(s) by which fibrin(ogen) or its derivatives increase tumor cell success remain to be established. In this regard, important lingering questions include: 1) What is the relative importance of soluble fibrinogen, fibrin polymerization, and fibrin degradation products? 2) Does fibrinogen serve as a "molecular bridge" between tumor and endothelial cells through specific integrin and non-integrin receptors? 3) Does fibrin(ogen) merely stabilize tumor cell association with the vessel wall, or does it shield tumor cells from immune surveillance mechanisms, support transendothelial cell migration, or provide some combination of benefits (and liabilities) to embolized tumor cells? 4) What is(are) the role(s) of fibrinogen and platelet interactions in determining tumor cell metastatic success?

Fibrinogen and tumor stroma formation

Fibrin deposition is a frequent feature of solid tumors and has been proposed to promote tumor stroma formation and angiogenesis. To test the hypothesis that fibrin(ogen) is important in tumor growth and angiogenesis, we subcutaneously injected a suspension of LLC cells into fibrinogen-deficient and control animals. All mice were found to develop palpable tumors within a few days of tumor cell injection, regardless of animal genotype. In addition, no differences in solid tumor growth rates were found over an observation period of two weeks [9]. Similarly, no genotype-related differences were found in the microscopically measured size distribution of individual pulmonary metastatic foci 3 weeks after intravenous injection of either LLC or B16 tumor cells. These findings are consistent with the hypothesis that fibrin(ogen) alters metastatic potential by a mechanism that is unrelated to growth of established tumors.

A detailed analysis of the impact of fibrinogen on tumor stroma has not yet been made, but preliminary microscopic analyses of LLC- and B16-derived primary (subcutaneous) tumors and secondary pulmonary metastatic foci reveal no obvious differences in overall tumor architecture in fibrinogen-deficient and control animals. Furthermore, preliminary studies highlighting primary tumor vasculature by immunohistochemistry using an anti-PECAM antibody suggest that there is substantial tumor angiogenesis in fibrinogen-deficient mice and that any differences in tumor vasculature are likely to be very subtle. However, detailed qualitative studies (e.g., vascular branching and patency within tumors) and quantitative studies (e.g., vessel diameters and density) are still required.

Fibrinogen and spontaneous metastasis.

One limitation of experimental metastasis studies is that they do not provide any information about earlier phases in the metastatic process (i.e., the time frame in which cells must dissociate from the primary tumor mass, invade through extracellular matrices and tissue barriers, penetrate vascular basement membranes, and enter the circulation). A priori, the impact of fibrinogen deficiency on spontaneous tumor metastasis could not be predicted based on experimental metastasis assays, and, in principle, the results could be opposite of those observed in experimental metastasis tests. Conceivably, the absence of fibrin matrices within primary tumor tissue might promote the escape of tumor cells by removing at least one physical barrier that must be negotiated in order to enter the circulation. On the other hand, the absence of fibrin in and around solid tumors might impede early steps in the metastatic process by destabilizing the tumor stroma or removing an important (provisional) matrix component that supports tumor cell migration. Indeed, fibrin might be an asset to tumor cells at certain stages of the metastatic process and a liability at other stages. Fortunately, the fact that fibrinogen did not appear to have a major impact on solid tumor growth in the tumor models employed in our studies permitted a meaningful analysis of the role of this specific hemostatic factor in the development of spontaneous metastases. Like earlier hematogenous metastasis results, fibrinogen deficiency was found to greatly diminish, but does not eliminate, the spontaneous metastasis of solid subcutaneous LLC tumors. In these studies, we transplanted LLC cells into the subcutis of fibrinogen-deficient mice and control animals, and twelve days later (median tumor weight of 420 mg) we either: i) surgically removed the primary tumors with electrocautery to minimize bleeding, or ii) controlled the primary tumors by local electron beam irradiation. Two weeks after primary tumor control, mice were sacrificed and surface pulmonary metastases counted. Both methods of local control resulted in a significant diminution in spontaneous metastases in fibrinogen-deficient mice relative to control animals. Both surgery and radiotherapy were used as complementary approaches to eliminate the primary tumor growth in order to control experimental concerns unique to each approach. For example, although tissue borders were apparently clear of tumor cells in the surgical procedure, the surgical approach raises the issue of whether tumor cell shedding lead to genotype-dependent differences in tumor dissemination. Similarly, with the tumor irradiation approach, local inflammatory or immunological responses to the necrotic tissue may lead to a genotype-dependent difference in the formation of metastatic lesions. However, the results of these studies show that regardless of the means used to experimentally eliminate the primary tumor, fibrinogen deficiency appears to diminish the formation of metastatic foci.

The Fibrinogen–Platelet Axis and Tumor Dissemination.

Multiple lines of evidence support the concept that platelet-tumor cell interaction and tumor cell-induced platelet activation are important in hematogenous metastasis. Double-label fluorescence microscopy studies [12] have provided direct evidence of tumor cell-platelet interactions in vivo. Furthermore, pharmacological diminution in either platelet number or platelet activation pathways using antibodies and other agents (e.g., thrombin inhibitors) have been frequently shown to diminish tumor cell metastasis [13,14]. In addition, anti-adhesion receptor antibodies focusing on either platelet cell surface receptors (e.g., the fibrinogen-binding integrin, $\alpha IIb\beta 3$) or tumor cell adhesion molecules (e.g., the fibrinogen-binding adhesion molecules, ICAM-1) have been shown to be effective anti-metastatic agents [15]. Nevertheless, the putative role of platelets in metastasis has remained uncertain because the available data is based solely on studies using anti-platelet agents that either are not specific, are short lasting, or have potential secondary pharmacological effects that obscure interpretation. Furthermore, there has been a distinct absence of supporting studies that provide clear insights into mechanism(s). Proposed hypotheses include: 1) platelets support tumor cell arrest, 2) platelet-derived growth factors support the proliferation of tumor cells, 3) platelets potentiate endothelial cell retraction and subsequent tumor cell extravasation, and 4) tumor cell-associated platelets provide a "cloaking device" that blocks natural killer cell-mediated elimination of tumor cells. These concepts are not mutually exclusive and the relative merit of each (and every) theory remains unclear. Clearly an important focus for future studies will be to define the interplay between fibrinogen, platelets and tumor cells in establishing metastatic disease foci. This line of inquiry will be aided by the availability of mouse lines with specific deficits in platelet receptor-fibrinogen interactions [16] and other profound deficits in platelet function [17,18].

References

1. Dvorak HF: Tumors: wounds that do not heal. Similarities between tumor stroma generation and wound healing. N Engl J Med. 1986;315:1650-1659.
2. Shapiro RL, Duquette JG, Roses DF, Nunes I, Harris MN, Kamino H, Wilson EL, Rifkin DB: Induction of primary cutaneous melanocytic neoplasms in urokinase-type plasminogen activator (uPA)-deficient and wild-type mice: cellular blue nevi invade but do not progress to malignant melanoma in uPA-deficient animals. Cancer Res. 1996;56:3597-3604.
3. Eitzman DT, Krauss JC, Shen T, Cui J, Ginsburg: Lack of plasminogen activator inhibitor-1 effect in a transgenic mouse model of metastatic melanoma. Blood. 1996;87:4718-4722.
4. Sabapathy KT, Pepper MS, Kiefer F, Mohle-Steinlein U, Tacchini-Cottier F, Fetka I, Breier G, Risau W, Carmeliet P, Montesano R, Wagner EF: Polyoma middle T-induced vascular tumor formation: the role of the plasminogen activator/ plasmin system. J Cell Biol. 1997;137:953-963.
5. Bugge TH, Kombrinck KW, Xiao Q, Holmback K, Daugherty CC, Witte DP, Degen JL: Growth and dissemination of Lewis lung carcinoma in plasminogen-deficient mice. Blood. 1997;90:4522-4531.
6. Bugge TH, Lund LR, Kombrinck KK, Nielsen BS, Holmback K, Drew AF, Flick MJ, Witte DP, Dano K, Degen JL: Reduced metastasis of Polyoma virus middle T antigen-induced mammary cancer in plasminogen-deficient mice. Oncogene. 1998;16:3097-3104.
7. Bajou K, Noel A, Gerard RD, Masson V, Brunner N, Holst-Hansen C, Skobe M, Fusenig NE, Carmeliet P, Collen D, Foidart JM: Absence of host plasminogen activator inhibitor 1 prevents cancer invasion and vascularization. Nat Med. 1998;4:923-928.
8. Gutierrez LS, Schulman A, Brito-Robinson T, Noria F, Ploplis VA, Castellino FJ: Tumor development is retarded in mice lacking the gene for urokinase-type plasminogen activator or its inhibitor, plasminogen activator inhibitor-1. Cancer Res. 2000;60:5839-5847.
9. Palumbo JS, Kombrinck KW, Drew AF, Grimes TS, Kiser JH, Degen JL, Bugge TH: Fibrinogen is an important determinant of the metastatic potential of circulating tumor cells. Blood. 2000;96:3302-3309.
10. Bajou K, Masson V, Gerard RD, Schmitt PM, Albert V, Praus M, Lund LR, Frandsen TL, Brunner N, Dano K, Fusenig NE, Weidle U, Carmeliet G, Loskutoff D, Collen D, Carmeliet P, Foidart JM, Noel A: The plasminogen activator inhibitor PAI-1 controls in vivo tumor vascularization by interaction with proteases, not vitronectin. Implications for antiangiogenic strategies. J Cell Biol. 2001;152:777-784.
11. Frandsen TL, Holst-Hansen C, Nielsen BS, Christensen IJ, Nyengaard JR, Carmeliet P, Brunner N: Direct evidence of the importance of stromal urokinase plasminogen activator (uPA) in the growth of an experimental human breast cancer using a combined uPA gene-disrupted and immunodeficient xenograft model. Cancer Res. 2001;61:532-537.
12. Borsig L, Wong R, Feramisco J, Nadeau DR, Varki NM, Varki A: Heparin and cancer revisited: Mechanistic connections involving platelets, P-selectin, carcinoma mucins, and tumor metastasis. Proc Natl Acad Sci U S A. 2001;98:3352-3357.
13. Honn KV, Tang DG, Crissman JD: Platelets and cancer metastasis: a causal relationship? Cancer Metastasis Rev. 1992;11:325-351.
14. Nieswandt B, Hafner M, Echtenacher B, Mannel DN: Lysis of tumor cells by natural killer cells in mice is impeded by platelets. Cancer Res. 1999;59:1295-1300.
15. Nierodzik ML, Klepfish A, Karpatkin S: Role of platelets, thrombin, integrin IIb-IIIa, fibronectin and von Willebrand factor on tumor adhesion in vitro and metastasis in vivo. Thromb Haemost. 1995;74:282-290.
16. Holmback K, Danton MJ, Suh TT, Daugherty CC, Degen JL: Impaired platelet aggregation and sustained bleeding in mice lacking the fibrinogen motif bound by integrin alpha IIb beta 3. Embo J. 1996;15:5760-5771.
17. Offermanns S, Toombs CF, Hu YH, Simon MI: Defective platelet activation in G alpha(q)-deficient mice. Nature. 1997;389:183-186.
18. Shivdasani RA, Rosenblatt MF, Zucker-Franklin D, Jackson CW, Hunt P, Saris CJ, Orkin SH: Transcription factor NF-E2 is required for platelet formation. independent of the actions of thrombopoietin/MGDF in megakaryocyte development. Cell. 1995;81:695-704.

Hæmostasis

Lectures

Haemostasis 2001;31(suppl. 1):16-20

Angiogenesis

Relationship of blood clotting and tumor angiogenesis

FREDERICK R RICKLES
The George Washington University Medical Center and the Children's National Medical Center; Washington, DC, USA

Tissue factor (TF), the 47 KDa transmembrane protein activator of blood coagulation, has additional biologic functions, including the promotion of tumor angiogenesis [1-3] and cell adhesion [4]. The bifunctional properties of TF as both a pro-clotting and an adhesive and pro-angiogenic protein probably contributes to its important role in the enhancement of tumor growth and metastasis [3,5]. This relationship of blood clotting to tumor angiogenesis extends further in the hemostatic system to the platelet release reaction, soluble clotting factors and their inhibitors, cross-linked fibrin and, finally to the fibrinolytic cascade, a rich source of both positive and negative regulators of angiogenesis [6]. Perhaps, given the important role of platelet, clotting and fibrinolytic proteins in the maintenance of the hemostatic plug, and tissue and vascular repair processes, it should not surprise us that one or more of these proteins can also serve to either enhance or inhibit new vessel formation [Figure; Reference 7].

As has been reviewed in preceding papers, tumor cells themselves possess a variety of procoagulant properties, including the constitutive, cell surface expression of TF, the secretion of the cysteine protease, cancer procoagulant (CP), that directly cleaves factor X, and procoagulant cytokines such as IL-1, IL-8 and vascular endothelial growth factor (VEGF). Tumor cell VEGF is chemotactic for both macrophages and endothelial cells and activates TF in both types of cell. Tumor cells also activate platelets and, via integrin expression, form adhesive interactions with platelets and the endothelium of blood vessels. Tumor cell interaction with the vessel wall reduces endothelial cell secretion of tissue plasminogen activator (TPA) and expression of thrombomodulin (TM), and increases endothelial cell synthesis of plasminogen activator inhibitor (PAI-1). Finally, substantial experimental evidence supports the presence of increased numbers of activated monocytes/macrophages in the circulation of cancer patients and in proximity to growing tumors. These antigen-processing cells express TF on their surface, presumably as part of the host immune response to the tumor and/or in response to secretion of tumor products. Tumor-associated macrophages have been shown to assemble the entire coagulation cascade and form cross-linked fibrin on their surface in apposition to growing tumor. The activation of coagulation in the tumor microenvironment, which routinely spills into the circulation of cancer patients, rendering them "hypercoagulable", may be a primitive effort on the part of the host to limit the spread of tumor cells [3]. Macrophage TF expression in cancer patients (measured in cultured peripheral blood monocytes) correlates significantly with plasma levels of the thrombin-induced, fibrinogen activation peptide, fibrinopeptide A (FPA). Although correlation never proves causation, it is notable that cross-linked fibrin (XLF) can be co-localized with TF in both tumor-associated macrophages and within the endothelium of tumor-associated blood vessels in human breast and lung cancer. The finding of TF expression in vascular endothelial cells (VECs) in proximity to or within a growing tumor lends further support for the concept that new vessels formed as a result of angiogenic signals generated by tumors may be more

KARGER
Fax +41 61 306 12 34
E-Mail karger@karger.ch
www.karger.com

0301-0147/00/0309/0001$17.50/0

Accessible online at:
www.karger.com/journals/hae

Frederick R. Rickles
The George Washington University
Ross Hall 712E - 2300 Eye St NW
Washington, DC 20037 USA
Tel: +1/202/994-2995 - Fax +1/202/994-0465
resfrr@gwia.gwumc.edu

susceptible to thrombogenesis. Further, this observation stimulated further exploration of a possible role for TF in the development of neoangiogenesis. Interleukin-8 is a potent pro-angiogenic cytokine elaborated by a variety of cells, including VECs. Cross-linked fibrin formed on the surface of VECs up-regulates the gene for IL-8 and induces the synthesis and release of increasing concentrations of functional IL-8 from VECs in a dose-dependent fashion. XLF also induces the expression of the TF gene in VECs at concentrations readily achievable in vivo and in the absence of thrombin. Therefore, it seems likely that multiple products of blood coagulation, including both thrombin and fibrin, can stimulate the activation and migration of endothelial cells (perhaps via IL-8 release) and induce a self-perpetuating system for further activation of blood coagulation (by induction of TF). Co-localization of TF and VEGF genes and functional antigens in situ in human lung and breast cancer cells further supports the potential for joint regulation of both clotting reactions and angiogenesis in human tumors [7,8].

A unifying hypothesis that could link the expression of TF and the development of new blood vessel formation in tumors was suggested by experiments in murine tumors described by Zhang and colleagues [1]. These investigators demonstrated that expression of VEGF in murine tumor cells was upregulated by transfection of the gene for TF into the cells. Furthermore, the level of the anti-angiogenic peptide thrombospondin varied inversely in the cells with the expression of TF. Once transplanted into a syngeneic murine recipient, tumors expressing high levels of the TF gene became highly vascularized. Neo-angiogenesis occurred in spite of maximal anticoagulation of the recipient mice or pretreatment of the tumor cells in vitro to minimize the potential for coagulation activation following transplantation. These results clearly suggested a new role for TF in the stimulation of angiogenesis, independent of its role as the primary trigger of blood coagulation. We extended these experiments to human breast and melanoma tumors grown as xenografts in immunodeficient mice. In 10 human breast cancer cell lines and 13 human melanoma cell lines, we demonstrated a strong correlation between levels of TF and VEGF generated in vitro ($r = 0.84$, $p < 0.0001$; $r = 0.94$, $p < 0.0001$, respectively) [2]. We selected, respectively, a high TF and VEGF producer (RPMI-7951) and a low producer (WM-115) melanoma cell line for further study.

Both the high producer and low producer cell lines generated tumors in SCID mice. The high producer cell lines generally resulted in highly vascular tumors within 8-10 weeks, as determined by immunohistochemical analysis with either anti-von Willebrand factor or anti-CD31 antibodies. Inoculation of SCID mice with the low producer cell lines resulted in rather avascular tumors on gross inspection with scant numbers of visible blood vessels by immunohistochemical analysis of at least 10, 200x microscopic fields by a blinded observer (RPMI-7951 = 17.3 ± 4.0 vs. WM-115 = 3.2 ± 2.2; $p = 0.01$) [2]. To test the hypothesis that this observed difference in vascularity in vivo between high TF-expressing and low TF-expressing tumors might be the result of molecular regulation of VEGF expression by TF, we transfected full-length TF cDNA in the sense orientation into another low producer melanoma cell line, HT-144 and analyzed the cells in vitro for both TF and VEGF production. Successful transfection of the full-length TF cDNA into the HT144 endogenous low producer cell line restored synthesis of both TF and VEGF to normal levels, supporting the hypothesis that TF somehow participates in the regulation of VEGF synthesis [2]. Consistent with data published by Bromberg and colleagues in a mouse tumor model after intravenous injection of melanoma cells [9], a TF mutant lacking the cytoplasmic domain (but retaining full procoagulant function) failed to sustain VEGF production in vitro or angiogenesis in vivo in our model [2]. In control experiments, VEGF transcription was fully restored in the cells with either the full-length TF sequence or with an extracellular domain mutant sequence ($Y^{157} \rightarrow A^{157}$ and $K^{159} \rightarrow A^{159}$), the latter of which prevents successful TF-mediated factor X activation by the cells [2]. These data indicate that the TF cytoplasmic tail is sufficient to induce VEGF transcription and that factor VIIa/factor X interactions are not required in this model. The in vitro observations were confirmed in vivo in xenogeneic tumors in nude mice, in which tumors resulting from the wild type cells were generally avascular and those resulting from the cells containing the full-length TF transfectant were replete with CD31+ blood vessels. Having demonstrated that TF can regulate VEGF production in vitro and in vivo, we began to develop a strategy for delivering inhibitors of both TF and VEGF production to tumor cells that might result ultimately in a novel therapeutic approach to cancer therapy.

Other groups have successfully targeted TF in both tumor cells and VECs in experimental approaches to model tumors [10-12]. Zhang and colleagues [10] and Huang et al. [11] developed novel strategies for targeting the tumor vasculature, taking some advantage of the apparently selective expression of TF in the neoangiogenic vessels of experimental murine tumors. Zhang et al. demonstrated that even in those tumors where the cancer cells themselves expressed little or no TF, the VECs expressed TF upon induction with tumor necrosis factor (TNF). TNF induction stimulated the production of fibrin in the vessels perfusing the tumor resulting in tumor necrosis. Blood flow was restored to the tumors with somatic gene transfer of anti-sense to TF. Huang et al. treated neuroblastomas in mice by intravenous adminis-tration of a bifunctional immunoconjugate consisting of a truncated, soluble form of TF (that retains only limited PCA) targeted with a monoclonal antibody to an expressed antigen specific for murine tumor endothelium [11]. This conjugate resulted in thrombosis of tumor vessels and complete tumor regression in 38% of the treated mice. A similar strategy as that employed by Huang et al. was employed successfully by Hu et al. [12], who regressed human melanoma in immunodeficient mice using an active site mutated factor VIIa conjugate that targeted TF in the endothelium of angiogenic vessels. We demonstrated previously that inactivated recombinant factor VIIa (rVIIai) is a specific and high affinity ligand for TF expressed on the surface of human tumor cells both in vitro and in situ. Factor VIIa mutated at the active site or inactivated with a tripeptide, chloromethyl ketone inhibitor retains its affinity for TF but is incapable of activating clotting. Factor VIIa binding to TF on cell surfaces also induces translocation of TF-VIIa complexes into caveolae, a phenomenon that is mediated equally well by rVIIai. We used rVIIai as a "Trojan Horse" to carry potential toxins into TF-bearing tumor cells and tumor-associated VECs. Curcumin [1,7-Bis(4-dydroxy-3methoxyphenyl)-1,6-heptadiene-3,5-dione], a major chemical component of the curry spice turmeric, has been found to have a variety of interesting biologic properties in various experimental systems. In particular curcumin blocks phorbol ester- and TNFα-induced TF synthesis by VECs by binding and inhibiting the action of the transcription factors NF-kB, AP-1 and Egr-1 [13,14] and curcumin inhibits angiogenesis in vivo [15]. In preliminary studies utilizing tumor cells and human VECs, we demonstrated that a series of synthetic curcumin analogs inhibit both TF and VEGF gene expression in vitro [16]. Studies are in progress to determine if one or more of the analogs linked to rVIIai can be utilized effectively to target TF and VEGF in tumor cells and tumor-associated blood vessels in vivo. It is our hope that this approach, which targets TF, might provide a bifunctional therapy for both the hypercoagulability and the excessive angiogenesis in cancer.

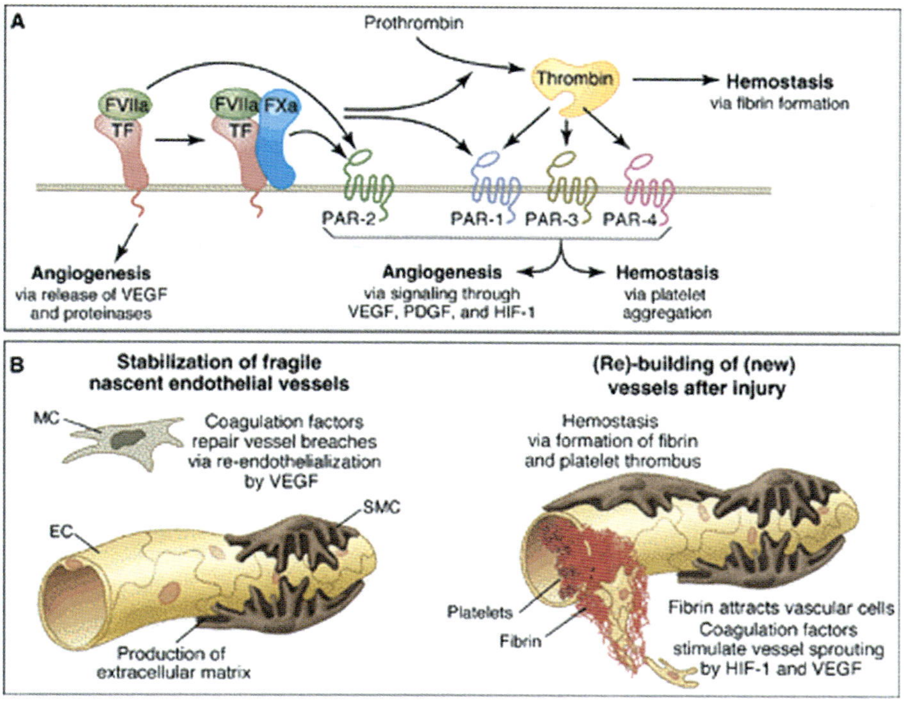

(A) *Initiation of coagulation by tissue factor/FVIIa sequentially generates FXa,thrombin, and fibrin —all essential for clot formation.Activation of PARs by thrombin stimulates platelet aggregation.Coagulation factors also induce angiogenic signaling in vascular cells.Arrows indicate interactions between receptors and their ligands.*

(B) *Possible coagulation factor involvement in angiogenesis and vessel stabilization. (Left)Fragile newly forming endothelial (EC)vessels are stabilized by recruitment of mesenchymal precursor cells (MC), which differentiate into contractile smooth muscle cells (SMC) and produce extracellular matrix (ECM). (Right)Upon vascular injury,coagulation stops bleeding (hemostasis)through formation of a fibrin and platelet thrombus.Coincidently, coagulation factors stimulate the repair of injured vessels and may contribute to the building of new vessels by activating HIF-1 and releasing VEGF.*

Fibrin provides a provisional matrix for migrating vascular cells during the formation of new blood vessels [Reprinted with permission from (Carmeliet P. Clotting factors build blood vessels. Science 2001;293:1602-1604). Copyright (2001) American Association for the Advancement of Science].

References

1. Zhang Y, Deng Y, Luther T, Muller M, Ziegler R, Waldherr R, Stern DM, Nawroth PP. Tissue factor controls the balance of angiogenic and antiangiogenic properties of tumor cells in mice. J Clin Invest 1994;94:1320-1327.
2. Abe K, Shoji M, Chen J, Bierhaus A, Danave I, Micko C, Casper K, Dillehay DL, Nawroth PP, Rickles FR. Regulation of vascular endothelial growth factor production and angiogenesis by the cytoplasmic tail of tissue factor. Proc Nat Acad Sci (USA) 1999;96:8663-8668.
3. Rickles FR, Levine M, Dvorak HB. Abnormalities of Hemostasis in Malignancy. In: Hemostasis and Thrombosis, 4th Edition. Eds: RW Colman, J Hirsh, VJ Marder, A Clowes and JN George. Lippincott Williams & Wilkins, Philadelphia, PA, Chapter 69, 2000, pp. 1132-1152.
4. Ott I, Fischer EG, Miyagi Y, Mueller BM, Ruf W. A role for tissue factor in cell adhesion and migration mediated by interaction with actin-binding protein 280. J Cell Biol 1998;140:1241-1253.
5. Rickles FR, Shoji M, Abe K. The role of the hemostatic system in tumor growth, metastasis and angiogenesis: tissue factor is a bifunctional molecule capable of inducing both fibrin deposition and angiogenesis in cancer. Int J Hematol 2001; 73:145-150.
6. Browder T, Folkman J, Pirie-Shepherd S. The hemostatic system as a regulator of angiogenesis. J Biolog Chem 2000;275:1521-1524.
7. Carmeliet P. Clotting factors build blood vessels. Science 2001;293:1602-1604.
8. Shoji M, Hancock WW, Abe K, et al. Activation of coagulation and angiogenesis in cancer. Immunohistochemical localization in situ of clotting proteins and VEGF in human cancers. Am J Pathol 1998;152:399-411.
9. Bromberg ME, Konigsberg WH, Madison JF, Pawashe A. Tissue factor promotes melanoma metastasis by a pathway independent of blood coagulation. Proc Nat Acad Sci (USA) 1995;92:8025-8029.
10. Zhang Y, Deng Y, Werndt T, et al. Intravenous somatic gene transfer with antisense tissue factor restores blood flow by reducing tumor necrosis factor-induced tissue factor expression and fibrin deposition in mouse meth A sarcomas. J Clin Invest 1996;97:2213-2224.
11. Huang X, Molema G, King S, Watkins L, Edgington TS, Thorpe PE. Tumor infarction in mice by antibody-directed targeting of tissue factor to tumor vasculature. Science 1997;275:547-555.
12. Hu Z, Sun Y, Garen A. Targeting tumor vasculature endothelial cells and tumor cells for immunotherapy of human melanoma in a mouse xenograft model. Proc Nat Acad Sci (USA), 1999;96:8161-8166.
13. Bierhaus A, Zhang Y, Quehenberger P, Luther T, Haase M, Muller, Mackman N, Ziegler R, Nawroth PP. The dietary pigment curcumin reduces endothelial tissue factor gene expression by inhibiting binding of AP-1 to the DNA and activation of NF-kappa B. Thromb Haemost 1997;77:772-782.
14. Pendurthi UR, Williams JT, Rao LVM. Inhibition of tissue factor gene activation in cultured endothelial cells by curcumin. Suppression of activation of transcription factors Egr-1, AP-1, and NF-kB. Arterioscl Thromb Vasc Biol 1997;17:3406-3413.
15. Arbiser JA, Klauber N, Rohan R, van Leeuwen R, Huang M-T, Fisher C, Flynn E, Byers HR. Curcumin is an in vivo inhibitor of angiogenesis. Molec Med 1998;4:376-383.
16. Adams BK, Davis MC, Ferstl EM, Snyder JP, Liotta DC, Rickles FR, Shoji M. Inhibition of tissue factor-mediated VEGF production and tumor cell growth by synthetic curcumin analogs. Blood (Suppl) 1999;94:12a (Abstract).

Hæmostasis

Lectures

Haemostasis 2001;31(suppl. 1):21-22

Targeted delivery of tissue factor to tumor neovasculature for cancer therapy

DARIO NERI
Department of Applied BioSciences, Swiss Federal Institute of Technology, Zurich (Switzerland)

Angiogenesis, i.e., the proliferation of new blood vessels from pre-existing ones, is an underlying process in many human diseases, including cancer, blinding ocular disorders and rheumatoid arthritis. The ability to selectively target and occlude neovasculature will be potentially useful in diagnosis and treatment of angiogenesis-related diseases.

A good-quality marker for both tumoural and non-tumoural neovasculature is the extra-domain B (ED-B) of fibronectin, a sequence of 91 aminoacids that can be inserted into the fibronectin molecule by a mechanism of alternative splicing.

To date, the production of monoclonal antibodies directly recognising the ED-B domain has not been possible using hybridoma technology, because of tolerance. In collaboration with Prof. Dr. Luciano Zardi (Istituto Nazionale per la Ricerca sul Cancro, Genova, Italy), we have overcome this problem using large synthetic antibody phage libraries, generating several high-affinity antibody fragments specific for fibronectin containing the ED-B domain, and mapping their epitope onto the three-dimensional structure of the antigen. These antibodies stain vascular structures in tumour sections and selectively target tumour neovasculature, as shown in tumour-bearing mice using infrared fluorescence and radioactive techniques. Increased binding affinity leads to improved targeting of tumoural angiogenesis, as demonstrated by biodistribution studies performed using the L19 antibody fragment with affinity for the ED-B domain in the picomolar range and L19 mutants with reduced affinity.

The L19 antibody, chemically coupled to a photosensitiser and irradiated with red light, mediates the complete and selective occlusion of ocular neovasculature, as demonstrated in a rabbit model of ocular angiogenesis.

A fusion protein, consisting of the L19 antibody fused to the extracellular domain of tissue factor, mediates the complete and selective infarction of three different types of solid tumours in mice. At the highest doses administered, complete tumour eradication was observed

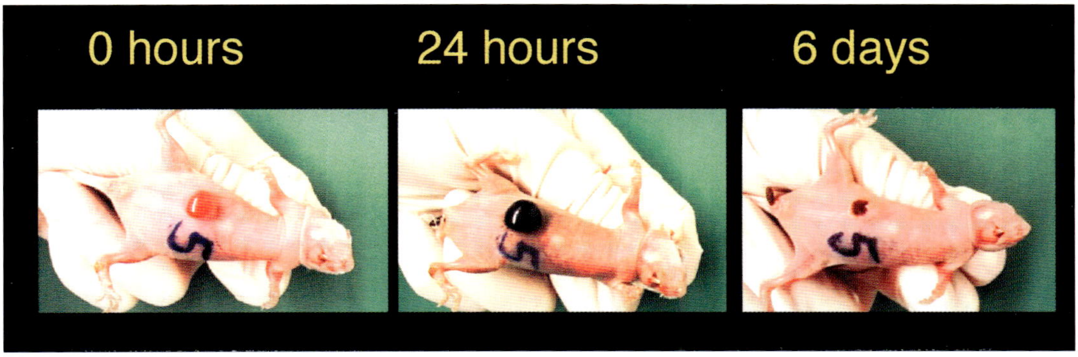

Legend: complete eradication of a F9 murine teratocarcinoma by intravenous injection of the L19-tissue factor fusion protein.

KARGER
Fax +41 61 306 12 34
E-Mail karger@karger.ch
www.karger.com

0301-0147/00/0309/0001$17.50/0

Accessible online at:
www.karger.com/journals/hae

Dario Neri
Department of Applied Biosciences - Swiss Federal Institute of Technology Zurich
Irchel Y36 M14 - Winterthurerstr. 190
CH-8057 ZURICH - SWITZERLAND
Tel. +41/1/6356063/6356082 - Fax +41/1/6356886
neri@pharma.anbi.ethz.ch

in 30% of the mice treated, without apparent side effects. Even more impressive results were obtained when the L19-tissue factor fusion protein was administered in combination with chemotherapeutic agents.
These results are of therapeutic relevance, since the ED-B domain of fibronectin, a naturally-occurring marker of angiogenesis identical in mouse and man, is expressed in the majority of aggressive solid tumours, but is undetectable in normal vessels and tissues.

References

1. Carnemolla, B., Neri, D., Castellani, P., Leprini, A., Neri, G., Pini, A., Winter, G. and Zardi, L. Phage antibodies with pan-species recognition of the oncofoetal angiogenesis marker fibronectin ED-B domain. Int. J. Cancer 1996; 68, 397-405.
2. D. Neri, B.Carnemolla, A. Nissim, E. Balza, A. Leprini, G. Querze', A. Pini, L. Tarli, C. Halin, P. Neri, L. Zardi, G. Winter. Targeting by affinity-matured recombinant antibody fragments of an angiogenesis associated fibronectin isoform. Nature Biotechnology 1997; 15, 1271-1275.
3. L. Pini, F. Viti, A. Santucci, B. Carnemolla, L. Zardi, P. Neri, D. Neri. Design and use of a phage-display library: human antibodies with subnanomolar affinity against a marker of angiogenesis eluted from a two-dimensional gel. J. Biol. Chem. 1998; 273, 21769-21776.
4. P. Kirkham, D. Neri and G. Winter. Towards the design of an antibody that recognises a given epitope. J. Mol. Biol. 1999, 285, 909-915.
5. F. Viti, L. Tarli, L. Giovannoni, L. Zardi, D. Neri. Binding affinity and valence determine the tumour targeting performance of anti-angiogenesis antibodies. Cancer Res. 1999; 59, 347-352.
6. Carnemolla, P.Castellani, M. Ponassi, L. Borsi, S. Urbini, G. Nicolo', A. Dorcaratto, G. Viale, G. Winter, D. Neri and L. Zardi. Identification of a glioblastoma associated TN-C isoform by a high affinity recombinant antibody. Am. J. Pathol. 1999; 154, 1345-1352.
7. L. Tarli, E. Balza, F. Viti, L. Borsi, P.Castellani, D. Berndorff, L. Dinkelborg, D. Neri, L. Zardi. A high-affinity human antibody that targets tumoural blood vessels. Blood 1999; 94, 192-198.
8. M. Birchler, F. Viti, L. Zardi, B. Spiess, D. Neri. Selective targeting and photocoagulation of ocular angiogenesis mediated by a phage-derived recombinant antibody. Nature Biotechnol. 1999; 17, 984-988.
9. F. Viti, F. Nilsson, S. Demartis, A. Huber, D. Neri. Design and use of phage display libraries, for the selection of antibodies and enzymes. Methods in Enzymology 2000; 326, 480-505.
10. F. Viti, M. Bumke, M. Silacci, L. Zardi, D. Neri. A strategy for the identification of differentially expressed proteins secreted by fibroblasts. Chimia 2000; 54, 678-682.
11. F. Nilsson, H. Kosmehl, L. Zardi, D. Neri. Targeted delivery of tissue factor to the ED-B domain of fibronectin, a marker of angiogenesis, mediates the infarction of solid tumours in mice, Cancer Res. 2001, 61, 711-716.
12. C.Halin, D. Neri. Antibody-based targeting of angiogenesis" Crit. Rev. Ther. Drug Carrier Syst. 2001; in press.
13. L. Giovannoni, F. Viti, L. Zardi, D. Neri. Isolation of anti-angiogenesis antibodies from a large combinatorial repertoire by colony filter screening. Nucleic Ac. Res. 2001; 29, No.5, e27.
14. S. Demartis, L. Tarli, L. Borsi, L. Zardi, D. Neri. In vivo targeting of tumour neo-vasculature by a radiohalogenated human antibody fragment specific for the ED-B domain of fibronectin. Eur. J. Nucl. Med. 2001; 28, 534-539.
15. C. Halin, L. Zardi, D. Neri. Antibody-based targeting of angiogenesis. News Physiol. Sci. 2001; 16, 191-194.

Hæmostasis

Lectures

Haemostasis 2001;31(suppl. 1):23-24

Thrombospondin-1: an inhibitor of angiogenesis

GIULIA TARABOLETTI
Mario Negri Institute for Pharmacological Research, Bergamo, Italy

Tumor angiogenesis is sustained by an increased production of angiogenic factors accompanied by a decreased production of inhibitors. Among the latter, thrombospondin -1 (TSP-1) is considered one of the chief physiological controllers of angiogenesis.

TSP-1 is a secreted trimeric 450 kDa glycoprotein, released by activated platelets and produced by different cell types, including tumor cells, endothelial cells, fibroblasts, and inflammatory cells. TSP-1 is a matricellular protein, namely a non-structural component of the extracellular matrix, which affects cell functions by modulating cell-matrix interaction [1]. The matricellular proteins present a modular structure, as they are composed by a series of distinct structural domains, each endowed with different (even opposite) activities. The TSP-1 modules can interact with several matrix components, cell receptors, soluble growth factors and proteolytic enzymes, therefore conferring to the molecule a high functional complexity.

Given these premises, it is not surprising that the role of TSP-1 in angiogenesis and tumor progression is multifaceted, and not yet completely understood [1-3]. TSP-1 is considered one of the main inhibitors of angiogenesis, as indicated by the evidence that TSP-1 inhibited angiogenesis induced by several factors in vitro and in vivo. Moreover, in experimental models as well as in clinical studies, the loss of TSP-1 production was associated with the acquisition of an angiogenic phenotype and with tumor progression, while restoration of TSP-1 production prevented angiogenesis and reduced tumor growth. It has been demonstrated that domains within the 140 kDa, carboxyterminal fragment mediate the antiangiogenic activities of TSP-1.

However, other studies aimed at clarifying the role of TSP-1 in angiogenesis have shown that TSP-1 was also able to stimulate microvessel formation in rat aorta explants and pro-angiogenic activities in endothelial cells such as endothelial cell adhesion, motility, invasion and production of matrix metallo-proteinases [1-4]. We have demonstrated that a domain within the aminoterminal, heparin-binding region of the molecule mediates these proangiogenic activities of TSP-1 [5]. Other endogenous inhibitors of angiogenesis are fragments of larger molecules (e.g. angiostatin and endostatin), however, the case of TSP-1 is particular since it acts as a source of both positive and negative smaller mediators of angiogenesis. TSP-1 hence represents a new class of dual regulators of angiogenesis whose activity depends not only on the presence of the molecule, but on which domain is available/functional.

Environmental condition as well as genetic alterations directly affect the production of angiogenesis regulatory factors by tumor cells. TSP-1 has been one of the firstly described examples of how oncogenes and tumor suppressor genes can directly control the production of endogenous inhibitors of angiogenesis [6]. TSP-1 production is stimulated by the tumor suppressor gene wt p53 [7] as well as by Rb, PTEN, and nm23, and inhibited by oncogenes, such as v-myc, c-jun, v-src, and polyoma virus middle T oncogene [6]. We have recently described that the production of TSP-1 by tumor cells and their overall angiogenic potential is also controlled by p73, another member of the p53 family [8].

The mechanisms at the basis of the antiangiogenic activity of TSP-1 have only partially been clarified. CD36, one of the TSP-1 receptors, has been described to mediate the antiangiogenic activity of TSP-1 [9], although a growing body of evidence suggests that other mechanisms are involved. We previously reported that TSP-1 binds to the angiogenic factor basic fibroblast growth factor (bFGF or FGF-2) [10]. TSP-1 also binds to other heparin-binding angiogenic factors, including VEGF, HGF/SF, PDGF and the HIV-1 product Tat. We have therefore hypothesized that the direct interaction of TSP-1 with angiogenic factors might affect their activity, and may thus

KARGER
Fax +41 61 306 12 34
E-Mail karger@karger.ch
www.karger.com

0301-0147/00/0309/0001$17.50/0

Accessible online at:
www.karger.com/journals/hae

Giulia Taraboletti
Mario Negri Institute for Pharmacological Research
Via Gavazzeni, 11 - 24125 BERGAMO ITALY
Tel. +39/035/319888 - Fax +39/035/319331
taraboletti@marionegri.it

represent a mechanism of the antiangiogenic activity of TSP-1. Heparin-binding angiogenic factors, including FGF-2, bind with high affinity to heparan sulfate proteoglycans (HSPG) of both the cell surface - where they mediate interaction with high affinity receptors and internalization - and the extracellular matrix - where they store the growth factors in a silent form. The release of active angiogenic factors from the matrix represents an important mechanism of the onset of tumor angiogenesis. Since TSP-1 binding to FGF-2 is inhibited by heparin, we have investigated whether TSP-1 might affect the interaction of angiogenic factors with HSPG.

We have found that TSP-1 prevented the binding of FGF-2 to its low affinity receptors on endothelial cells, and reduced the internalization of the growth factor. Furthermore, soluble TSP-1 dose dependently prevented the binding of labeled FGF-2 to the extracellular matrix, and caused the release of ECM-associated FGF-2. FGF-2 was released from the matrix by TSP-1 as a complex FGF/TSP and was not able to induce endothelial cell proliferation.

The inhibition of growth factor interaction with HSPG in the extracellular matrix by TSP-1 was not restricted to FGF-2. Other heparin-binding angiogenic factors, which bind to TSP-1, were affected: TSP-1 also inhibited the binding of VEGF and HGF/SF to the matrix and caused their release from the matrix.

We have identified the fragment of TSP-1 responsible for these functions: the 140 kDa, carboxyterminal fragment of the molecule, known for its antiangiogenic activity - but not the proangiogenic 25 kDa heparin binding fragment -, contains the binding site for FGF-2, prevents FGF-2 binding to low affinity receptor on the cell surface and to the extracellular matrix, and cause the release of FGF-2 from the matrix. Our study shows that TSP-1 regulates the interaction of angiogenic factors with the HSPG associated to both the cell surface and the matrix. This could contribute to the antiangiogenic activity of TSP-1.

References

1. Bornstein P. Thrombospondins as matricellular modulators of cell functions. J Clin Invest 2001; 107: 929-934, 2001
2. Roberts DD. Regulation of tumor growth and metastasis by thrombospondin-1. FASEB J 1996;10:1183-1191.
3. Tuszynski GP, Nicosia RF. The role of thrombospondin-1 in tumor progression and angiogenesis. BioEssays 1996;18:71-76.
4. Taraboletti G., et al. Platelet thrombospondin modulates endothelial cell adhesion, motility and growth: a potential angiogenesis regulatory factor. J. Cell Biol., 111: 765-772, 1990.
5. Taraboletti G., et al. The heparin binding 25 kDa fragment of thrombospondin-1 promotes angiogenesis and modulates gelatinase and TIMP-2 production in endothelial cells. FASEB J, 2000; 14: 1674-1676.
6. Bouck, N. How tumors become angiogenic. Adv. Cancer Res. 1996; 69: 135-174.
7. Dameron K.M, et al. Control of angiogenesis in fibroblasts by p53 regulation of thrombospondin-1. Science 1994; 265: 1582-1584.
8. Vikhanskaya F, Bani MR, Borsotti P, Ghilardi C, Ceruti R, Ghisleni G, Marabese M, Giavazzi R, Broggini M and Taraboletti G. p73 overexpression increases VEGF and reduces thrombospondin-1 production: implications for tumor angiogenesis. Oncogene, in press.
9. Dawson, D.W., Pearce, S.F.A., Zhong, R., Silverstein, R.L., Frazier, W.A., and Bouck, N.P. CD36 mediates the in vitro inhibitory effects of thrombospondin-1 on endothelial cells. J. Cell Biol. 1997; 138: 707-717.
10. Taraboletti G.,et al. The 140-kDa antiangiogenic fragment of thrombospondin-1 binds to basic fibroblast growth factor. Cell Growth Differ 1997; 8: 471-479.

Hæmostasis

Lectures

Haemostasis 2001;31(suppl. 1):25-29

Inhibition of angiogenesis with heparin?

SUSANNE M. SMORENBURG
Department of Cell Biology and Histology, Academic Medical Center, University of Amsterdam, Amsterdam, The Netherlands

In summary, TSP-1 is a complex regulator of angionesis, as i) it contains both pro- and anti-angiogenic domains; and ii) its antiangiogenic activity can be achieved through different mechanisms. Future studies will clarify the processes that control the production, availability and activity of the angiogenesis regulatory sequences of TSP-1.
Patients with malignant diseases are at increased risk of venous thromboembolic complications. As a result, many cancer patients are treated with antithrombotic drugs, including unfractionated heparin and low molecular weight heparin. Interestingly, clinical studies have indicated that treatment with low molecular weight heparin can prolong survival of cancer patients [1]. On the other hand, experimental studies have shown that heparins can affect various steps in tumor growth and metastasis in a complex and unpredictable manner (see [2] for review).

Heparins are members of a family of polysaccharides, the glycosaminoglycans. Unfractionated heparin is isolated and purified from animal tissues (porcine intestinal mucosa or bovine lung) and has a mean molecular weight of 12-15 kD. Low molecular weight heparin consists of fragments of unfractionated heparin, produced by controlled enzymatic or chemical depolymerization, with a mean molecular weight of approx. 5 kD and less than 18 saccharide units. Heparins exert their anticoagulant effects by activating the physiological coagulation inhibitor antithrombin that neutralizes many of the serine proteases involved in the coagulation system, particularly thrombin and activated factor X. Besides binding to antithrombin, unfractionated heparin, and to a lesser extent low molecular weight heparin, bind to a wide range of other proteins and molecules by electrostatic interactions with its polyanionic groups. These interactions are modulated by physiochemical properties of heparin such as sequence, degree of sulfation, charge distribution, overall charge and molecular size. Consequently, heparins have a wide variety of biological activities other than their anticoagulant effects which may interfere with the malignant process.

Experimental studies have shown that heparins can affect angiogenesis, an important process in tumor progression. Angiogenesis, the formation of new blood vessels from existing vessels, supports the expansion of solid tumors and facilitates the escape of cancer cells into the circulation and thus metastasis [3]. Angiogenesis is driven by microvascular endothelial cells, that when activated by angiogenic growth factors degrade their basement membrane, migrate into the interstitial matrix, proliferate, and form new capillary-like tubular structures [4].
Heparins can affect angiogenesis in various ways. In 1983, Folkman and colleagues reported that angiogenesis was inhibited by treatment with combinations of unfractionated heparin and corticosteroids, whereas treatment with corticosteroids alone had no or little effect [5]. They also showed that tumor growth was arrested in mouse models of cancer by combined treatment with heparins and corticosteroids and that metastasis to the lungs was prevented. Nevertheless, the mechanism by which this combinational therapy inhibited angiogenesis was unknown and the results could not be reproduced with heparins manufactured by other companies. Moreover, studies in other laboratories reported inconclusive results of this combined treatment [6-8].
Other studies have reported that heparins affect angionesis without addition of corticosteroids, by interaction with angiogenic growth factors. Tumors release a number of angiogenic factors, such as vascular endothelial growth factor (VEGF), fibroblast growth factors and scatter factor [9]. The angiogenic

KARGER
Fax +41 61 306 12 34
E-Mail karger@karger.ch
www.karger.com

0301-0147/00/0309/0001$17.50/0

Accessible online at:
www.karger.com/journals/hae

Susanne M. Smorenburg
Department of Vascular Medicine F4-227 - Academic Medical Center
Meibergdreef 9 - 1105 AZ Amsterdam - THE NETHERLANDS
Tel. +31/20/5665976 - Fax +31/20/6968833
s.m.smorenburg@amc.uva.nl

factors can bind to heparan sulfate proteoglycans that are present on endothelial cell surfaces and in the extracellular matrix. Binding to heparan sulfates results in stabilization and relative inactivation of these growth factors as well as prevention of their diffusion and proteolytic degradation [10]. Therefore, it has been proposed that heparan sulfates in the extracellular matrix have an important role in storage of growth factors that can be released when needed to exert their effects immediately upon release [11]. Soluble heparins compete with heparin sulfates for binding of growth factors and other molecules, and may thus cause release of these proteins from the extracellular matrix [12]. In man, therapeutic dosages of unfractionated heparin can indeed cause increased plasma levels of growth factors, such as scatter factor and basic fibroblast growth factor (bFGF) [13, 14].

Heparins or heparan sulfates are also considered to have a crucial role in modulation of binding of growth factors to their high affinity receptors. This phenomenon has been thoroughly studied for bFGF [15]. bFGF activates its high affinity receptors on endothelial cells by inducing dimerization of its receptors. Multivalent complexes of bFGF and heparins or heparan sulfates promote bFGF receptor activation by dimerization even stronger [15]. Interestingly, it has been reported that low molecular weight heparin, in contrast to unfractionated heparin, can hinder binding of growth factors to their high affinity receptors as a consequence of its smaller size. Indeed, *in vitro* heparin fragments with a size of less than 18 saccharide residues reduced activity of VEGF, whereas activity of bFGF was inhibited by fragments with a size of less than 10 saccharide residues [16, 17].

In a recent *in vitro* study, we investigated the effects of unfractionated heparin and low molecular weight heparin on proliferation of human microvascular endothelial cells and human umbilical vein endothelial cells [18]. In contrast to previous studies, both unfractionated heparin and low molecular weight heparin inhibited VEGF- and bFGF- mediated proliferation of microvascular endothelial cells in a concentration-dependent way, whereas proliferation of human umbilical vein endothelial cells was not affected by either agent. Because angiogenesis is especially driven by microvascular endothelial cells, this effect is probably relevant for tumor neovascularization. In this study, we also evaluated other steps in the process of angiogenesis that may be affected by heparins, in particular interactions of microvascular endothelial cells with the matrix that they invade. For these experiments, human microvascular endothelial cells were seeded on top of a fibrin matrix, that was altered by addition of either low molecular weight heparin or unfractionated heparin during polymerization. The cells were induced by angiogenic growth factors to form capillary-like tubular structures. Turbidity measurements and electron microscopy showed that the presence of low molecular weight heparin during polymerization of the fibrin matrix led to a more transparent and rigid network of thin fibrin bundles, whereas the presence of unfractionated heparin resulted in a more opaque malleable network of thick fibrin fibers. The formation of capillary-like tubular structures was retarded in matrices polymerized in the presence of low molecular weight heparin, whereas matrices polymerized in the presence of unfractionated heparin facilitated tubular structure formation. These data show that heparins not only affect proliferation of endothelial cells by interaction with growth factors, but also affect angiogenesis *in vitro* by altering structural and mechanical properties of the fibrin network. Whereas structural alterations of the fibrin matrix by unfractionated heparin enhances invasion of the matrix by capillary-forming endothelial cells, low molecular weight heparin reduces it.

Fibrin is a major component of the initial stroma of several tumor types and provides a scaffold during invasion of both cancer and endothelial cells. Therefore, it is conceivable that unfractionated heparin and low molecular weight heparin also affect *in vivo* angiogenesis in tumors differently. However, *in vivo* studies of the effects of heparins on tumor-associated angiogenesis are limited. Nevertheless, various experimental studies have shown that unfractionated heparin does not affect growth of subcutaneously implanted primary tumors, whereas it either reduces, increases or does not affect spontaneous metastasis (Table 1) [19-31]. Although effects of heparin on tumor-associated angiogenesis per se were not evaluated, the results of these studies indicate that potential effects of unfractionated heparin on angiogenesis do not result in altered primary tumor growth. To investigate more precisely the hypothesis that unfractionated heparin and low molecular weight heparin differently affect tumor-associated angiogenesis, we compared quantitatively the effects of treatment with unfractionated heparin, low molecular weight heparin or placebo on the development of experimentally induced colon carcinoma metastases in livers and highly vascularized osteosarcomas of rats [32, 33]. Notwithstanding the therapeutic plasma levels of heparins that were obtained, both colon cancer metastasis in liver and the growth of osteosarcomas were not affected by either treatment. Number, size and differentiation grade of metastases or osteosarcomas were comparable in all treatment groups. Moreover, intra-tumor vessel density was not affected by either unfractionated or low molecular weight heparin in both experiments.

On the basis of these recent studies, we like to conlude that heparins may affect angiogenesis *in vitro* in various ways. Moreover, the effects of unfractionated heparin on *in vitro* angiogenesis differ from those of low molecular weight heparin. However, thus far, there is no convincing evidence from animal studies that heparins also affect tumor-associated angiogenesis *in vivo*. Most likely because of the wide variety of activities of heparins and thus the complex effects on various steps in angiogenesis and carcinogenesis, the ultimate effect of heparin-treatment on these processes remains unpredictable.

Table 1.* Effects of unfractionated heparin on subcutaneously implanted tumors and their spontaneous metastasis.

Reference	Tumor type	Primary tumor	Spontaneous metastases
Antachopoulos et al. [19]	(Human) Colon carcinoma (nude mice)	=	=
Drago et al. [20]	Prostate carcinoma	=	↓ (various organs)
Hagmar [21]	Rhabdomyosarcoma	=	= (lungs)
Hagmar [22]	Rhabdomyosarcoma	=	↑ (lungs) = (lymphnodes)
Hagmar [23]	Rhabdomyosarcoma	=	↑ (lungs)
Lee et al. [24]	Mammary carcinoma	=	↓ (lungs)
Lee et al. [25]	Mammary carcinoma	=	↓ (lungs)
Maat and Hilgard [26]	Lewis lung carcinoma	=	= (lungs)
	Melanoma	=	= (lungs)
Milas et al. [27]	Fibrosarcoma	=	↓ (lungs)
	Mammary carcinoma	=	↓ (lungs)
Ohkoshi et al. [28]	Squamous cell carcinoma		
Owen [29]	Walker sarcoma	=	
Retik et al. [30]	Sarcoma (T-241)	=	↑ (lungs)
	Sarcoma (DBA-49)	=	= (lungs)
Wood jr et al. [31]	Lewis lung carcinoma	=	↓ (lungs)

* Table published in: Smorenburg & van Noorden [2].

References

1. Hettiarachchi RJK, Smorenburg SM, Ginsberg J, et al. Do heparins do more than just treat thrombosis? The influence of heparins on cancer spread. Thromb Haemost 1999; 82: 947-952.
2. Smorenburg SM, van Noorden CJF. The complex effects of heparins on cancer progression and metastasis in experimental studies. Pharmacol Rev 2001; 53: 93-105.
3. Hanahan D, Folkman J. Patterns and emerging mechanisms of the angiogenic switch during tumorigenesis. Cell 1996; 86:353-64.
4. Folkman J, Watson K, Ingber D et al. Induction of angiogenesis during the transition from hyperplasia to neoplasia. Nature 1989; 339: 58-61.
5. Folkman J, Langer R, Linhardt RJ et al. Angiogenesis inhibition and tumor regression caused by heparin or a heparin fragment in the presence of cortisone. Science 1983; 221: 719-725.
6. Penhaligon M, Camplejohn RS. Combination heparin plus cortisone treatment of two transplanted tumors in C3H/He mice. J Natl Cancer Inst 1985; 74: 869-873.
7. Ziche M, Ruggiero M, Pasquali F et al. Effects of cortisone with and without heparin on angiogenesis induced by prostaglandin E1 and by S180 cells, and on growth of murine transplantable tumours. Int J Cancer 1985; 35: 549-552.
8. Teale DM, Underwood JC, Potter CW et al. Therapy of spontaneously metastatic HSV-2 induced hamster tumours with cortisone acetate administered with or without heparin. Eur J Cancer Clin Oncol 1987; 23: 3-100.
9. Kumar R, Kuniyasu H, Bucana CD et al. Spatial and temporal expression of angiogenic molecules during tumor growth and progression. Oncol Res 1998; 10: 301-311.
10. Rusnati M, Presta M. Interaction of angiogenic basic fibroblast growth factor with endothelial cell heparan sulfate proteoglycans. Biological implications in neovascularization. Int J Clin Lab Res 1996; 26: 15-23.
11. Colin S, Jeanny JC, Mascarelli F et al. In vivo involvement of heparan sulfate proteoglycan in the bioavailability, internalization, and catabolism of exogenous basic fibroblast growth factor. Mol Pharmacol 1999; 55: 74-82.
12. Vlodavsky I, Ishai-Michaeli R, Mohsen M et al. Modulation of neovascularization and metastasis by species of heparin. Adv Exp Med Biol 1992; 313: 317-327.
13. Taniguchi T, Toi M, Tominaga T. Rapid induction of hepatocyte growth factor by heparin. Lancet 1994; 344: 470
14. Yamazaki H, Oi H, Matsushita M et al. Heparin induces rapid and remarkable elevation of hepatocyte growth factor/scatter factor during trans arterial embolization of renal cell carcinoma. Anticancer Res 1997; 17: 1435-1437.
15. Schlessinger J, Lax I, Lemmon M. Regulation of growth factor activation by proteoglycans: what is the role of the low affinity receptors? Cell 1995; 83: 357-360.
16. Jayson GC, Gallagher JT. Heparin oligosaccharides: inhibitors of the biological activity of bFGF on Caco-2 cells. Br J Cancer 1997; 75: 9-16.
17. Soker S, Goldstaub D, Svahn CM et al. Variations in the size and sulfation of heparin modulate the effect of heparin on the binding of VEGF165 to its receptors. Biochem Biophys Res Commun 1994; 203: 1339-1347.
18. Collen A, Smorenburg SM, Peters E et al. Unfractionated and low molecular weight heparin affect fibrin structure and angiogenesis in vitro. Cancer Res 2000; 60: 6196-6200.
19. Antachopoulos CT, Gagos S, Iliopoulos DC et al. Low-dose heparin treatment does not inhibit SW480 human colon cancer growth and metastasis in vivo. In Vivo 1996; 10: 527-531.
20. Drago JR, Weed P, Fralisch A. The evaluation of heparin in control of metastasis of Nb rat androgen-insensitive prostate carcinoma. Anticancer Res 1984; 4: 171-172.
21. Hagmar B. Effect of heparin, epsilon-aminocaproic acid and coumarin on tumour growth and spontaneous metastasis formation. Pathol Eur 1968; 3: 622-630.
22. Hagmar B. Effect of heparin, coumarin and -aminocaproic acid (EACA) on spontaneous metastasis formation. Influence on the moment of metastasis formation. Possible cytotoxic effect of heparin and coumarin in blood. Pathol Eur 1969; 4: 283-292.
23. Hagmar B. Tumour growth and spontaneous metastasis spread in two syngeneic systems. Acta Pathol Microbiol Scand 1970; 78: 131-142.

24. Lee AE, Rogers LA, Jeffery RE et al. Comparison of metastatic cell lines derived from a murine mammary tumour, and reduction of metastasis by heparin. Clin Exp Metastasis 1988; 6: 463-471.
25. Lee AE, Rogers LA, Longcroft JM et al. Reduction of metastasis in a murine mammary tumour model by heparin and polyinosinic-polycytidylic acid. Clin Exp Metastasis 1990; 8: 165-171.
26. Maat B, Hilgard P. Anticoagulants and experimental metastases-evaluation of antimetastatic effects in different model systems. J Cancer Res Clin Oncol 1981; 101: 275-283.
27. Milas L, Hunter N, Basic I. Treatment with cortisone plus heparin or hexuronyl hexoaminoglycan sulfates of murine tumors and their lung deposits. Clin Exp Metastasis 1985; 3: 247-255.
28. Ohkoshi M, Akagawa T, Nakajima M. Effects of serine protease inhibitor FOY-305 and heparin on the growth of squamous cell carcinoma. Anticancer Res 1993; 13: 963-966.
29. Owen jr CA. Anticoagulant treatment of rats with Walker 256 carcinosarcoma. J Cancer Res Clin Oncol 1982; 104: 191-193.
30. Retik AB, Arons MS, Ketcham AS et al. The effect of heparin on primary tumors and metastases. J Surg Res 1962; 11: 49-53.
31. Wood jr S, Holyoke ED, Yardley JH. Mechanisms of metastasis production by blood-born cancer cells. Canad Canc Conf 1961; 4: 167-223.
32. Smorenburg SM, Vink R, te Lintelo M et al. In vivo treatment of rats with unfractionated heparin or low molecular weight heparin does not affect experimentally induced colon carcinoma metastasis. Clin Exp Metastasis 1999; 17: 451-456.
33. Smorenburg SM, Botman M, Mulder WJ et al. Treatment with unfractionated heparin or low molecular weight heparin does not affect growth of sarcomas and tumor-associated angiogenesis in an experimental rat model. In: Smorenburg SM. Heparins, Cancer and Thrombosis. Clinical and Experimental studies. Thesis. Amsterdam, The Netherlands, Thela Thesis, 2000.

Hæmostasis

Lectures

Haemostasis 2001;31(suppl. 1):30-31

The human vascular mapping project.
Selection and utilization of Molecules for Tumor endothelial targeting.

WADIH ARAP, RENATA PASQUALINI*
M.D. Anderson Cancer Center, University of Texas, Houston, TX, U.S.A.
Amsterdam, The Netherlands

We are creating the first molecular map of the human vasculature. The map comprises ligand-receptor pairs located on the cells forming blood vessels of both normal and diseased tissues, including tumors. Our unique screening strategy enables organ- and tumor-homing probes to be isolated based on a human functional screening, the ability to home selectively to human blood vessels of an organ, tumor, or defined site. In addition, our imaging technology affords an anatomical and cellular context to the expression and accessibility of targeted probes to identified receptors. These unique receptor locations are referred to as "vascular zip codes." The mapping of blood vessel addresses in normal or diseased tissues will enable the targeting and manipulation of such receptors for therapeutic, diagnostic, or imaging purposes. It will also help optimize delivery tools including peptides, antibodies, and chemical analogs. The identification of unique vascular zip codes will make targeted medicine possible. We are creating this ligand-receptor pair map based on technologies that incorporate in vivo phage display, high throughput DNA sequencing, high throughput receptor identification and cloning, in vivo imaging, and bioinformatics. We are also creating a searchable database of the ligand-receptor pairs constituting the map. Our purpose is to develop safe and efficacious clinical products using the knowledge we possess about the molecular diversity of blood vessels.

The *in vivo* selection method we developed is based on the identification of peptides that home to specific vascular beds. They are selected after intravenous administration of a phage display random peptide library [1]. We have established tools for tissue-specific targeting of normal blood vessels [2,3] and angiogenesis-related targeting of tumor blood vessels [4,8]. Targeting peptides have been used by several groups as carriers to guide the delivery of cytotoxic drugs [5], pro-apoptotic peptides [8], metalloprotease inhibitors [7], cytokines [9], fluorophores [10], and genes [11]. Generally, coupling to homing peptides yields targeted compounds that are more effective and less toxic than the parental compound [5,8,9]. Moreover, vascular receptors corresponding to the selected peptides have been identified in blood vessels of normal organs [14] and in tumor blood vessels [13,14]. Taken together, these results show that this technology can be used to generate targeted therapies.

Vascular targeting will enable the guided delivery of therapeutics, diagnostics, and imaging agents to vascular addresses of normal organs and to angiogenic addresses of tumors or other diseased tissues. The value of vascular markers over tissue specific markers is clear: circulating probes have direct access to markers selectively expressed on cells forming blood vessels. Such probes do not have access to specific tissue markers outside of vessels unless they first leak out of the blood vessel. Further, it is clear from our work, and the work of others, that the gene expression profiles of the cells forming blood vessels is largely inducible rather than constitutive. Therefore, molecular addresses on blood vessels can change in disease, and in vivo screening strategies provide better information than in vitro screening strategies. Since we are interested in accelerating drug discovery in human disease, it follows that human in vivo screening is the most predictive model for any drug candidate.

We are pursuing a three-pronged strategy. We will (1) determine human vascular zip codes for the most

KARGER

Fax +41 61 306 12 34
E-Mail karger@karger.ch
www.karger.com

0301-0147/00/0309/0001$17.50/0

Accessible online at:
www.karger.com/journals/hae

Wadih Arap
The University of Texas - M.D. Anderson Cancer Center
1515 Holcome Bld, Box #427 - Houston, Texas 77030 - USA
Tel. +1/713/7923871 - Fax +1/713/7452999
warap@notes.mdacc.tmc.edu - warap@mail.mdanderson.org

promising lead candidates, (2) give access to the human vascular zip code data base to others in the scientific community, and (3) develop our own lead therapy candidates. We are the only group in the world with access to data from the human vasculature in vivo. In general terms, any compound, agent, drug, vector, or device can be screened for its ability to home, target, or modulate a receptor in a given site in the human vasculature. This quick screen mechanism in humans--rather than in models--will directly address questions regarding activity and species specificity of a vascular targeted therapy. Access to validated, unique ligand-receptor pairs in the human vasculature may enable our group and our drug discovery collaborators to rule out potential drug candidate failures and identify potential drug candidate winners much earlier in the drug

References

1. Pasqualini, R., Arap, W., Rajotte, D. & Ruoslahti, E. In Vivo Phage Display; in Phage Display: A Laboratory Manual (C. F. Barbas III, D. R. Burton, J. K. Scott & G. J. Silverman, eds.) Chapter 22, pp. 1-24 (Cold Spring Harbor Laboratory Press, New York, NY, 2000).
2. Pasqualini, R. & Ruoslahti, E. Organ targeting in vivo using phage display peptide libraries. Nature 380, 364-366 (1996).
3. Rajotte, D. et al. Molecular heterogeneity of the vascular endothelium revealed by in vivo phage display. J. Clin. Invest. 102, 430-437 (1998).
4. Pasqualini, R., Koivunen, E. & Ruoslahti, E. αv integrins as receptors for tumor targeting by circulating ligands. Nature Biotechnol. 15, 542-546 (1997).
5. Arap, W., Pasqualini, R. & Ruoslahti, E. Cancer treatment by targeted drug delivery to tumor vasculature in a mouse model. Science 279, 377-380 (1998).
6. Burg, M. A., Pasqualini, R., Arap, W., Ruoslahti, E. & Stallcup, W. B. NG2 proteoglycan-binding peptides target tumor neovasculature. Cancer Res. 59, 2869-2874 (1999).
7. Koivunen, E. et al. Tumor targeting with a selective gelatinase inhibitor. Nature Biotechnol. 17, 768-774 (1999).
8. Ellerby, H. M. et al. Anti-cancer activity of targeted pro-apoptotic peptides. Nature Med. 5, 1032-1038 (1999).
9. Curnis, F. et al. Enhancement of tumor necrosis factor a antitumor immunotherapeutic properties by targeted delivery to aminopeptidase N (CD13). Nature Biotechnol. 18, 1185-1190 (2000).
10. Hong, F. D. & Clayman, G. L. Isolation of a peptide for targeted drug delivery into human head and neck solid tumors. Cancer Res. 60, 6551-6556 (2000).
11. Trepel, M., Grifman, M., Weitzman, M. D. & Pasqualini, R. Molecular adaptors for vascular-targeted adenoviral gene delivery. Hum. Gene Ther. 11, 1971-1981 (2000).
12. Rajotte, D. & Ruoslahti, E. Membrane dipeptidase is the receptor for a lung-targeting peptide identified by in vivo phage display. J. Biol. Chem. 274, 11593-11598 (1999).
13. Pasqualini, R. et al. Aminopeptidase N is a receptor for tumor-homing peptides and a target for inhibiting angiogenesis. Cancer Res. 60, 722-727 (2000).
14. Bhagwat, S. V. et al. CD13/APN is activated by angiogenic signals and is essential for capillary tube formation. Blood 97, 652-659 (2001).
15. Kolonin, M. G., Pasqualini, R. & Arap, W. Molecular addresses in blood vessels as targets for therapy. Curr. Opin. Chem. Biol. 5, 308-313 (2001).

Hæmostasis

Lectures

Haemostasis 2001;31(suppl. 1):32-33

Epidemiological aspects of thrombosis in cancer

Venous thromboembolism and occult malignancy: an historical perspective

HANS MARTIN MB OTTEN [1], MARTIN H PRINS [2]
1 Department of Internal Medicine,
2 Department of Clinical Epidemiology and Medical Technology Assessment, Academic Hospital Maastricht, University of Maastricht, The Netherlands

Armand Trousseau (1801-1867), was the first to write about an association between venous thromboembolism (VTE) and malignancy [1]. Subsequently the term Trousseau's syndrome was coined to venous thrombosis as a presenting feature of neoplastic disease. A close analysis of his lecture would indicate that (considering the limited availability of diagnostic tools in his time) concurrent phlegmasia indicated that malignancy was the underlying disorder that caused the symptoms. Hereafter several lectures and studies have been published confirming the relation between thrombosis and cancer, but not occult cancer [2,3,4]. The first ones to report the observation of VTE as sign of truly occult malignancy were Illtyd James and Matheson in 1935 [5].
Up to 1951 an association between occult cancer and VTE was based only on case reports and necropsies, not quite the evidence physicians would currently require for guiding their clinical practice. In 1951 the first cohort study was published, a retrospective investigation on the prognosis and morbidity of thrombophlebitis. [6] Unfortunately, the authors did not have objective tests ad their disposal to confirm the diagnosis of deep venous thrombosis. In addition, 27% of the patients were lost for follow-up. Nevertheless, of the 67 patients with VTE, 6 (9%) appeared to have an underlying, occult malignancy. Hereafter some studies were published on the relation of occult malignancy and venous thrombosis [7,8,9]. However, it took another 30 years for the first proper cohort study to appear [10].

Because of the association between cancer and VTE, investigators became interested in the prevalence of concomitant cancer in (idiopathic) VTE. In patients presenting with VTE, the prevalence of concomitant cancer, defined as cancer not known before VTE and discovered by routine investigation (history taking, physical examination, simple laboratory tests like ESR, whole blood count, liver and kidney function tests, urinalysis and chest X-ray) varies considerably between the studies. This variation might relate to the depth of the routine examinations and to the characteristics of the included patients. Another part of the explanation is the variability of definition used for secondary thrombosis and differences in threshold of suspicion. It seems that some of the differences can also be explained by the age of the patients. The studies of Ahmed et al. and Subira et al. that both found a zero prevalence contained almost exclusively patients younger than 40 years [11,12]. They did not find any concomitant cancer in this age category. There are 7 other studies that investigate the prevalence of concomitant cancer and differentiated between secondary and idiopathic VTE. In these studies risk of concomitant cancer was increased among patients with idiopathic VTE by a factor 3 to 19. The larger series report a significant increased risk by a factor 3 to 4. The prevalence of concomitant cancer in patients with secondary VTE was

KARGER
Fax +41 61 306 12 34
E-Mail karger@karger.ch
www.karger.com

0301-0147/00/0309/0001$17.50/0

Accessible online at:
www.karger.com/journals/hae

Martin H. Prins
Department of Clinical Epidemiology and Medical Technology Assessment
Academic Hospital Maastricht - University of Maastricht
P.Debyelaan 5800 - P.B. 5800
6202 AZ Maastricht - THE NETHERLANDS
mh.prins@epid.unimaas.nl

low and in general comparable with the 2 to 3 % prevalence expected in the general population after middle age [13].
It is reasonable to consider malignancies detected up to 3 years after a VTE, not known before VTE and not detected by routine investigations at time of VTE, to be occult at the time of VTE. In total 17 cohort and 2 population based studies investigated the prevalence of occult cancer. The prevalence of occult cancer in patients with idiopathic VTE, of 40 years or more, is roughly between 4 and 10%. This figure is in all studies, that allow comparison, higher than in patients with secondary thrombosis. It is interesting to note that three studies with extensive screening procedures for cancer at the time of thrombosis tend towards a lower incidence of a diagnosis of cancer later on.

References

1 Trousseau A. Plegmasia alba dolens. In: Bailliere J.B. editor. Clinique Médicale de l'Hotel-Dieu de Paris, 2nd ed. Paris: J.B. Bailliere et fils. 1865;3:654-712.
2 Haward W. Phlebitis and thrombosis. Lancet 1906;1:650-5.
3 Barker NW. Thrombophlebitis complicating infectious and systemic diseases. Proc Staff Meet Mayo Clin 1936;11:513-7.
4 Hoerr SO, Harper JR. On peripheral thrombophlebitis. JAMA. 1957;164:2033-4.
5 Illtyd James TGI, Matheson NM. Thrombo-phlebitis in cancer. Practitioner 1935;134:683-4.
6 Ackerman RF, Estes JE. Prognosis in idiopathic thrombophlebitis. Ann Intern Med. 1951;34:902-10.
7 Woolling KR, Shick RM. Thrombophlebitis: a possible clue to cryptic malignant lesions. Proc Staff Meet Mayo Clin. 1956;31(8):227-33.
8 Anlyan WG, Shingleton WW, Delaughter GD. Significance of idiopathic venous thrombosis and hidden cancer. JAMA. 1956;161(10):964-6.
9 Lieberman JS, Borrero J, Urdaneta E, Wright IS. Thrombophlebitis and cancer. JAMA. 1961;177(8):542-5.
10 Gore JM, Appelbaum JS, Greene HL, Dexter L, Dalen JE. Occult cancer in patients with acute pulmonary embolism. Ann Intern Med. 1982;96:556-60.
11 Ahmed Z, Mohyuddin Z. Deep vein thrombosis as a predictor of cancer. Angiology. 1996;47:2615.
12 Subirà M, Mateo J, Souto JC, Altés A, Fontcuberta J. Lack of association between venous thrombosis and subsequent malignancy in a retrospective cohort study in young patients. Am J Hematol. 1999;60:181-4.
13 Coebergh JWW. Incidence and prognosis of cancer in The Netherlands: studies based on cancer registries. [dissertation] Rotterdam Univ. 1991:191-5.

Hæmostasis

Lectures

Haemostasis 2001;31(suppl. 1):34-36

Screening for cancer in patients with venous thromboembolism

HENRIK TOFT SØRENSEN
Department of Clinical Epidemiology, Aarhus University Hospital and Aalborg Hospital

The association between cancer and venous thromboembolism is well known, and over 100 years ago Trousseau reported cases of episodic migratory thrombophlebitis in patients with cancer [1]. Occasionally, the thromboembolic event occurs before the diagnosis of cancer, and it has been suggested, based on small studies, that venous thromboembolism may be a predictor of subsequent cancer in the years afterwards. However, only few studies have been large enough to identify the cancer sites most associated with thrombosis. Many aspects of these relations are poorly understood.

Risk of cancer after venous thromboembolism

Recently, two large registry based Scandinavian follow-up studies have provided clear evidence of an association between deep venous thromboembolism and the development of cancer [2,3]. The studies made it possible to get information about cancer site, specific risk and in the Danish study also the extent of the disease and prognosis; elements that are important for considering screening. Baron et al used the Swedish In Patient Register to identification of 61,998 patients with venous thromboembolism without a previous cancer admitted to hospitals in Sweden between 1965 and 1983 [2]. The data were linked to the nationwide Cancer Registry of the total population and the cancer incidence was assessed and compared with the expected cancer cases. The patients had a mean age of 63.9 years; 51% were male. The mean year of admission for thromboembolism was 1978. At the time of thromboembolic admission or during the first year of follow-up, 2,509 cancers gave a standardized incidence rate ratio (SIR) of 4.4 (95% CI: 4.2-4.6). The SIR for polycythaemia vera was 12.9. The SIRs for cancers of the liver, pancreas, ovary and brain exceeded 5.0. The risk was significantly higher among patients younger than 65 years of age than among patients who are 65 years or older [3].

A similar Danish record linkage study was based on 15,348 patients with deep venous thromboembolism and 11,305 patients with pulmonary embolism identified in the Danish Registry of patients established in 1977 [3]. 99.4% of all discharges from Danish medical hospitals are recorded here from January 1977 to December 1992. All members of the study cohorts were linked through their civil registry numbers to the nationwide Cause of Death Registry and Cancer Registry, which have kept records of all incident cases of cancer in Denmark since 1943 [3]. Both for patients with deep venous thromboembolism and for patients with pulmonary embolism the risk of cancer was increased during the first year of follow-up. There were strong associations in particular for cancer of the pancreas, ovary, primary hepatic cancer and brain. However, no associations were found for cancer of the breast, urinary bladder, rectum and malignant melanoma. 40% of the patients with cancer diagnosed during the first year of follow-up had distant metastasis (compared with 29% in a sex and age-matched population of patients with the same types of cancer), 25% regional spread, and 36% had no spread. Both the Swedish and Danish studies showed a 10 to 30% increased risk of cancer after the first year of follow-up [2,3]. Both studies were observational and the Danish study showed that many patients had distant metastasis at the time of diagnosis. Another Danish study showed that patients in whom cancer was diagnosed at the time of an episode of primary venous thromboembolism only 12% were alive after one year in contrast to 36% among cancer controls matched according to the type of cancer, age, sex and year of diagnosis and the survival was compared giving a mortality ratio of 2.5% (95% CI: 2.3-2.7) for the first year of follow-up period.

Screening for cancer in patients with VTE

Screening is here defined as identification of unrecognised cancer in patients with venous thromboembolism by history, physical examination, laboratory tests or other procedures. In our clinical

KARGER
Fax +41 61 306 12 34
E-Mail karger@karger.ch
www.karger.com

0301-0147/00/0309/0001$17.50/0

Accessible online at:
www.karger.com/journals/hae

Henrik Toft Sørensen
Department of Clinical Epidemiology - Aarhus University Hospital
Building 260 - Vennelyst Bld 6
DK- 8000 Aarhus C - DENMARK
Tel. +45/89/426077 - Fax +45/89/426110
hts@soci.au.dk

context the term screening is thus different from the original public health term, where a screening test is not intended to be diagnostic, but applied in patients with symptoms of disease.

When screening for occult cancer in patients with unexplained VTE one has to consider advantages and disadvantages in a screening programme. The main concern in setting up an extensive screening programme for all patients with unexplained VTE is that the cost-to-benefit ratio of such a screening programme has not been demonstrated definitively. In the evaluation of an extensive screening programme one must consider important matters such as i) the costs, ii) the accuracy of the screening method, iii) the potential benefit of early detection, and iv) the psychological and physical burdens of screening for an occult cancer, including false positive screens and "early" treatment that might be no better than later treatment. The costs and the discomfort related to an extensive screening procedure might be high, but it is probably more important to recognize that the extent and type of screening that should be offered patients with unexplained VTE is not easily determined. Effective screening tools with a sufficiently high sensitivity and specificity are thus not available for most of the cancers related to VTE, e.g. cancer of the liver, pancreas and ovary.

Furthermore, even though an extensive screening programme may identify early malignant disease, one must carefully consider whether the result favorably influences life expectancy and quality of life. Many patients with VTE have distant metastasis at the time of diagnosis, making it difficult to assess the benefit of searching for cancer, but extensive cancer screening of patients with VTE does not seem to be cost-effective. Thus, in our study, 26,600 persons would have to be screened for 304 excess cancers to be found [3]. Table 1 shows the number needed to screen in the Danish deep venous thrombosis cohort, which the only cohort restricted to patients with primary venous thrombosis. Lastly, the psychological and physical burdens of an extensive screening programme have to be considered. For example, a clinically silent malignant neoplasm may turn out to be inoperable or non-responsive to treatment, or a lesion suspected of being neoplastic may later be found to be non-malignant [5].

Even if cancers linked to unexplained VTE are detected with extensive screening methods like computer tomography scanning, ultrasonic scanning, gastrointestinal endoscopies, and detection of tumor markers, such procedures are only acceptable if they give potential gains in life expectancy in the long term. For the time being, there is still insufficient evidence of such a beneficial effect on survival with extensive screening programmes.

Table 1. Examples of the numbers needed to be screened (1/risk difference) in 15,348 patients with deep venous thrombosis.

	No. Observed	No. Expected	Risk Difference	Numbers needed to be screened
All neoplasms	390	181.5	205.5	74 patients
Pancreas	35	5.8	29.2	526 patients
Ovary	16	3.1	12.9	1,189 patients
Liver, primary	6	1.9	4.1	3,743 patients
Brain	10	3.3	6.7	2,291 patients
Non-Hodgkin's Lymphoma	10	3.5	6.5	2,361 patients
Esophagus	5	1.8	3.2	4,796 patients
Kidney	12	5.0	7.0	2,192 patients
Leukemia	11	4.4	6.6	2,325 patients
Prostate	58	13.7	44.3	346 patients

References

1. Phlegmasia alba dolens. In: Trousseau A. Lectures on clinical medicine, delivered at the Hotel-Dieu, Paris. Cormack JR, trans. London: New Sydenham Society, 1872:281-95.
2. Baron JA, Gridley G, Weiderpass E, et al. Venous thromboembolism and cancer. Lancet 1998; 351:1077-80. [Erratum, Lancet 2000; 355:758.]
3. Sørensen HF, Mellemkjær, Steffensen FH, et al. The risk of diagnosis of cancer after primary deep venous thrombosis or pulmonary embolism. N Engl J Med 1998; 338:1169-73.
4. Sørensen HT, Mellemkjær L, Olsen JH, et al. Prognosis of cancers associated with venous thromboembolism. N Engl J Med 2000; 343:1846-50.
5. Sørensen HT, Johnsen SP, Nørgård B, et al. Cancer and venous thromboembolism: a multidisciplinary approach. Submitted.

Hæmostasis

Lectures

Haemostasis 2001;31(suppl. 1):37-39

Idiopathic venous thromboembolism as a first manifestation of cancer

ANDREA PICCIOLI, PAOLO PRANDONI*
Department of Medical and Surgical Sciences, University of Padua, Italy

Abstract

Since Trousseau's time it has been documented the strong two-way relationship between cancer and venous thromboembolism (VTE). Moreover it has been clearly demonstrated that patients with a first episode of idiopathic VTE exhibit a higher risk of newly discovered cancer during follow-up when compared to those suffering from secondary VTE. The performance of a selected diagnostic work-up for cancer detection at the time of referral for index VTE in these patients appears to be capable to identify most of these malignancies and the earlier detection is likely to be associated with improved treatment possibilities and thus prognosis.

Article

For more than a century we have known that deep vein thrombosis and pulmonary embolism may be the presenting feature of an occult cancer [1]. Over time febrile research has clarified the consistency of the problem confirming this strong association and providing evidence that cancer and venous thromboembolism (VTE) are linked by a two-way clinical correlation. It has been in fact demonstrated that patients with cancer exhibit a higher incidence of VTE when compared to patients free from malignancy [2]. On the other hand, several reports have shown that the development of cancer during follow-up is more frequent in patients with confirmed VTE than in patients with suspected VTE but ruled out by objective tests [3]. Moreover it has been clearly demonstrated that among VTE patients the incidence of cancer in the follow-up is much higher in idiopathic VTE than in secondary one [4]. The assessment of this challenging topic has raised questions on its biological plausibility and has generated a long-standing debate on which could be the impact on patients care by screening for cancer patients presenting with a first episode of idiopathic VTE with no clinical complaint for underlying malignancy [5].

Pathogenetic bases accounting for the thrombotic disorders in cancer patients are complex and reflect the interaction of different mechanisms which are referred to as Virchow triad: they include hypercoagulability due to tumour cells activation of clotting, vessel wall injuries, and stasis. Main contributory causes to hypercoagulability include the ability of tumour cells and their products to interact with platelets, clotting system, as well as their interactions with endothelial surface and tumour associated macrophages causing an homeostatic imbalance between anticoagulant and procoagulant forces and resulting in a prothrombotic trigger [6].
Along with tumour-associated procoagulants the clotting system may be further perturbed by therapeutic cancer interventions or by the ability of cancer cells to injure vascular endothelium. Moreover venous stasis, commonly caused by immobilization due either to surgical procedures or worsening general conditions, venous obstruction and increased blood viscosity predispose to VTE by preventing activated coagulation factors from being cleared from the normal blood flow [7].

The great interest created on the subject together with the conclusive evidence of a strong association between idiopathic VTE and the risk of subsequent overt malignancy, have led the majority of the attending physicians to consider with suspect otherwise healthy patients presenting with an episode of idiopathic VTE.
It has been indeed shown that part of these cancers can be identified by routine assessment at the time of the thrombotic event. The prevalence of concomitant malignancy varies among literature data and this variation might be related once more to the different routine schedule adopted in singular hospital settings and to the characteristics of the investigated patients [8].
However, in apparently cancer-free patients at baseline, there remain approximately 10% incidence of subsequent overt malignancy in the following early period after the thrombotic event.
Despite this high incidence of cancer detection during the follow-up of these patients, whether to perform an extensive screening for malignancy in these patients is still

KARGER

Fax +41 61 306 12 34
E-Mail karger@karger.ch
www.karger.com

0301-0147/00/0309/0001$17.50/0

Accessible online at:
www.karger.com/journals/hae

Andrea Piccioli
Istituto di Clinica Medica II - Facoltà di Medicina e Chirurgia
Università degli Studi di Padova
Via Ospedale Civile, 105 - 35128 PADOVA - ITALY
andreapiccioli@libero.it

controversial and no standardized, prospectively validated guidelines are currently available on this subject. The lack of recommendations, often in contrast with physician consciousness of this real problem has produced over time a so called "singular hospital generated battery tests" for the detection of underlying cancer either on the basis of the available literature or guided by good clinical practice considering the prevalence of cancer types in the country. It has anyway to be pointed out that newly discovered cancers during follow-up of patients with VTE involve virtually all body systems and this pattern has to be taken in account when performing tests for cancer identification. Moreover, since extensive screening procedures are associated with high costs and also might result in some morbidity, they are acceptable only if they are cost-effective and if they have an impact on cancer related mortality.

To try to give a contribution to this important problem we have compared the strategy of an extensive screening versus no further testing for malignant diseases in a recently undertaken multicentre randomized clinical trial among 201 apparently cancer-free patients with an acute episode of idiopathic VTE in whom routine initial assessment did not reveal malignancy. Outcome of the study were cancer related mortality, recurrent malignancy, residual malignancy as well as to assess the sensitivity of the diagnostic work-up for occult malignancy (9). Out of 201 recruited patients, 99 were allocated to the extensive screening group, whereas the remaining 102 to the non further testing group. The extensive screening schedule is listed in table 1. All patients were followed up for two years. In the extensive screening group, 13 patients (13.1%) had the early detection of a histologically confirmed malignancy (in 10 cases revealed by CT scan of the abdomen and pelvis), and a further malignancy (1.0%) became apparent during follow-up. Therefore 13 of the 14 malignancies which became apparent in the extensive screening group were identified at the time of the screening, for a sensitivity of initial screening of 93% (95 CI, 66 to 100%). In the control group, a total of 10 (9.8%) malignancies became symptomatic during follow-up. Cancer related mortality occurred in 2 (2.0%) of the 99 patients in the extensive screening group as compared to 4 (3.9%) of the 102 control patients, for an absolute difference of 1.9% (95% CI: -5.5 to 10.9%). The cluster of cancer-related mortality, presence of objectively documented residual or recurrent malignancy occurred in 5 (5.1%) of the 99 patients in the extensive screening group as compared to 8 (7.9%) of the 102 control patients, for an absolute difference of 2.8% (95% CI: -6.3 to 13.4%) (10).

From all the above mentioned considerations the following issues can be highlighted:
1. Cancer and venous thromboembolism are linked together by a strong relationship.
2. Patients presenting with a first episode of idiopathic VTE carry a high risk of harbouring an underlying malignant disease, and should, therefore, be investigated with adequate battery tests.
3. A selected diagnostic work-up seems to be able to identify most of these cancers. The earlier detection might improve treatment possibilities and thus prognosis.

Table 1. Extensive screening programme in the SOMIT Study

Ultrasound of the abdomen and pelvis
CT-scan of the abdomen and pelvis
Gastroscopy or double contrast barium swallowing
Colonoscopy or sigmoidoscopy followed by barium enema
Haemoccult
Sputum citology and tumour markers (CEA, alpha-FP, Ca 125)
Mammography and Pap smear for women
Transabdominal Ultrasound of the prostate and PSA for men

References

1. Trousseau A. Phlegmasia alba dolens. In: Bailliere JB, Editor. Clinique Medicale de l'Hotel Dieu de Paris, 2nd Ed. 1865; 3 : 654-712.
2. Prandoni P, Piccioli A, Girolami A. Cancer and venous thromboembolism: an overview. Haematologica 1999; 84: 437-45.
3. Monreal M, Prandoni P. Venous thromboembolism as first manifestation of cancer. Semin Thromb Haemost 1999; 25: 131-6.
4. Piccioli A, Prandoni P. Venous thromboembolism as first manifestation of cancer. Acta Haematol 2001; 106: 13-17.
5. Prins MH, Lensing AWA. Idiopathic deep venous thrombosis: is a search for malignant disease justified? Arch Intern Med 1994; 154: 1310-2.
6. Rickles FR, Falanga A. Molecular basis for the relationship between thrombosis and cancer. Thromb Res 2001; 102 (Suppl): V215-24.
7. Piccioli A, Prandoni P, Ewnstein BM, Goldhaber SZ. Cancer and venous thromboembolism. Am Heart J 1996; 132: 850-5.
8. Otten HM, Prins MH. Venous thromboembolism and cancer. Thromb Res 2001; 102 (Suppl): V187-94.
9. Piccioli A, Lensing AWA, Prandoni P. Screening for occult malignancy in patients with idiopathic venous thromboembolism (SOMIT). Study Design. Thromb Haemost 1997 (Suppl): PS489.
10. Piccioli A, Lensing AWA, Prins MH, et al. Estensive screening for occult malignant disease in idiopathic venous thromboembolism. A prospective randomised clinical trial. Thromb Haemost 2001 (Suppl): OC900.

Hæmostasis

Lectures

Haemostasis 2001;31(suppl. 1):40-42

A number needed to screen and cost-effectiveness analysis of the SOMIT-data.

HANS-MARTIN MB. OTTEN [1], MARTIN H. PRINS [2].
1 Department of Internal Medicine, Academic Medical Center, in Amsterdam.
2 Department of Clinical Epidemiology, Academic Hospital Maastricht, in Maastricht.

Introduction

Only the last decades multiple reports showed the incidence of malignancy, in the 2 to 3 years after the first venous thromboembolism (VTE), appeared to be 7,5 % in patients with idiopathic VTE (IVTE), compared to 1,6 % in patients with a secondary VTE. [1] Taken into account the doubling time of cancer cells and the volume, needed to be detected, it is likely that the cancer was occult at the time of VTE. [2] The usefulness of screening procedures is not known. Recently the first prospective, randomized trial has been conducted comparing extensive screening procedures with basic screening in patients with IVTE. [3] The data were analyzed to determine the number needed to screen (NNS) to detect one additional case of cancer, for different diagnostic strategies. Next to the determination of the amount of patients harmed by each strategy, the costs of those strategies were calculated.

Methods

Study population

Calculations of number needed to screen analysis were based on the data from the SOMIT-study. [3] For details concerning the study population, definition of idiopathic VTE and methods of the SOMIT-study the reader is referred to the article of A. Piccioli et al.. Patients with first, idiopathic VTE, over 25 years old, were included. After basic screening for malignant disease was completed and negative, the patients were randomized. When allocated to the extensive screening group they were offered to undergo multiple procedures. (See Piccioli et al.) All patients had routine follow-up at 3, 12 and 24 months.

Number needed to screen analysis

The number of patients needed to screen, to detect one additional case of cancer was calculated by dividing the total number of patients in the extensively screened group, by the number of detected cases. This calculation was performed for several diagnostic strategies. When cancer was detected by more than one diagnostic procedure, it was only counted once. The number of patients evaluated further, due to abnormalities detected in the extensive screening, eventually because of a benign condition, was calculated for each diagnostic strategy, per cancer patient identified. We called it 'number harmed' (NH). This number was calculated by dividing the total number of patients evaluated further, eventually for a benign condition, by the number of detected cancer patients.

Decision Model

A decision model was developed representing 18 possible strategies for the diagnostic work-up for patients with IVTE. (See table 1) To be included, patients had to have a negative basic evaluation. Therefore basic evaluation was left out of the decision model. Sigmoidoscopy followed by barium enema was not considered in any model, because it is more expensive than colonoscopy and it lacks the possibility of taking biopsies proximal from the sigmoid.

Cost

Costs needed to detect one patient with a cancer were calculated. Costs were calculated from the perspective of the insurance system. Neither the costs made for initial treatment of the VTE, basic screening, and follow-up nor the costs related to the treatment of the cancer patients were taken into account.

For each strategy the costs of the screening tests were

KARGER
Fax +41 61 306 12 34
E-Mail karger@karger.ch
www.karger.com

0301-0147/00/0309/0001$17.50/0

Accessible online at:
www.karger.com/journals/hae

Hans-Martin MB. Otten
Academic Medical Center - Department of Internal Medicine
RM F4-222 - Meibergdreef 9 - 1105 AZ Amsterdam
THE NETHERLANDS
Tel. +31/20/5669111 - Fax +31/20/6919743
j.m.otten@amc.uva.nl

added up and multiplied by the number of patients who underwent the particular investigation. Patients with an abnormal test result were evaluated further. Per strategy the costs of those tests were calculated for each patient and were added up. These two figures were added up and were divided by the number of patients with cancer, detected by the strategy. The outcome represents the costs per patient with detected cancer. A common sense approach was used to determine the strategy of further evaluation, performed after an abnormal test result.
The costs were calculated in Euro's. (1 €= 0.92US$).

Results

Of the 99 patients in the extensive screening group, 14 had a histological confirmed malignancy within 2 years. Extensive screening was able to detect 13 of them.

Number needed to screen analysis

The results of the NNS and NH analysis are summarized in table 1. Most cancers were detected by means of Computer Tomography -abdomen/pelvis (CT- abd/pelv) with a low figure of false-positive cases. The addition of a Ultrasound (US)- abd/pelv or a gastroscopy to CT- abd/pelv yielded no additional cases, so the combination of those was not evaluated. The lowest NNS (7.6) was achieved by the combination of CT abd/pelv, mammography, sputum cytology and tumor markers. Unfortunately, for every cancer patient identified more than two were evaluated further for eventually a benign condition. The same problem accounts for all strategies that included tumor markers. The NNS of the combination CT abd/pelv and colonoscopy was 9.0 with a NH of 0.4. Part of the NH in this strategy is due to patients with a possible pre-malignant condition (tubular adenoma). The strategies using US-abd/pelv yielded a higher NNS (and a higher NH) in comparison to those using CT-abd/pelv. The strategies only using tumor markers performed comparable to those with US-abd/pelv.

Cost-effectiveness analysis

The mean difference between the calculations with and without the costs of the confirmation tests, was _ 204 (range 101-317). Most cost-effective was the performance of a CT-abd/pelv (€ 2,016). Least cost-effective was the strategy including only tumor markers together with hemoccult test (€ 42,407). The reason for this high figure was the amount of false positive results leading to further investigations. This applies for all strategies that included tumor markers and hemoccult tests. All strategies using colonoscopy, hemoccult test, tumor markers and ultrasound yielded costs, per cancer patient detected, above € 4,500. The addition of mammography or sputum cytology to CT-abd/pelv appeared to be somewhat less cost-effective (€ 2,124 respectively € 2,296) compared to CT-abd/pelv, due to small difference in NNS between these strategies. For the same reason, the combination of the three screening tests was more expensive (€ 2,371).

Discussion

In this analysis, the number needed to screen to detect one cancer patient in a group of patients with IVTE, was remarkable low, for several diagnostic strategies. Particularly the abdominal/pelvic CT-scan, with or without mammography and/or sputum cytology, yielded a NNS of 9.9 or less. These strategies appeared to result in few patients evaluated further due to false positive screening tests. All other strategies performed less because of higher NNS or NH. Most cost-effective strategy again was the CT-abd/pelv (€ 2,016). The strategies using colonoscopy, hemoccult test, tumor markers and/or ultrasound were 2.4 to 22.8 times as expensive as CT-abd/pelv, for each detected cancer patient.
This analysis has its limitations. The screened group consisted of only 99 patients. Earlier data showed that all kinds of malignancies are to be expected, solid and hematological. [4,5,6] So we should be suspicious to detect other malignancies as well. We hypothesized about the usefulness of a CT-scan of the chest in stead of sputum cytology. If the two patients with lung cancer were detected by means of CT-chest, with no false positive results, the costs per detected cancer patient would be € 3,475 for the combination with CT-abd/pelv and € 3,454 for the addition of mammography to that strategy. Furthermore the evaluation of patients with an abnormality in the initial screening was performed using common sense. It was impossible to make cost-effectiveness analysis concerning mortality. Due to circumstances explained in greater detail elsewhere the SOMIT-study was not able to detect a statistically significant difference in mortality between the screening and non-screening group. Nevertheless the extensive screening using CT-abd/pelv, sputum cytology and mammography was able to detect most malignancies in the patients with IVTE, at an acceptable rate. Whether this leads to a survival benefit in patients with IVTE remains to be investigated.

Table 1. Different strategies for the diagnostic work-up of patients with IVTE.

Strategy	NNS	NH	Costs in € per identified cancer patient
CT abd/pelv	9.9	0.1	2,016
CT + mammography	9.0	0.1	2,124
CT + sputum cytology	9.0	0.1	2,296
CT + mammography + sputum cytology	8.25	0.1	2,371
CT + markers	9.0	2.7	5,328
CT + mammography + sputum cytology + markers	7.6	2.4	6,251
CT + Hemoccult test	9.0	1.4	14,086
CT + Colonoscopy	9.0	0.4	5,141
US abd/pelv	19.8	0.2	5,098
US + mammography	16.5	0.2	4,782
US + sputum cytology	16.5	0.2	5,098
US + mammography + sputum cytology	14.1	0.2	4,827
US + markers	12.4	3.8	8,081
US + mammography + sputum cytology + markers	10.0	2.9	7,981
US + Colonoscopy	16.5	0.7	10,313
CEA. CA-125.α-FP. PSA and hemoccult test	16.5	7.8	42,407
CEA. CA-125.α-FP. PSA	16.5	5.2	13,281
CEA. CA-125.α-FP	19.8	4.6	14,798

NNS = Number needed to screen to identify one cancer patient.
NH = Number of patients harmed, to identify one cancer patient.

References

1 Otten HMMB, Prins M. Venous thromboembolism and occult malignancy. Thrombosis Research. 2001;102:V187-94.

2 Fingert HJ, Campisi J, Pardee AB. Cell proliferation and differentiation. In: Holland JF, Bast RC, Morton DL, Frei III E, Kufe DW, Weichselbaum RR, editors. Cancer Medicine. Baltimore: Williams and Wilkins. 1997. p. 3-18.

3 Piccioli A, Lensing AWA, Prins MH, Falanga A, Scannapieco L, Ieran M, Cigolini M, Bagatella P, Girolami A, Prandoni P, for the SOMIT Investigator Group. Extensive screening for occult malignant disease in idiopathic venous thromboembolism.
A prospective randomised clinical trial. Submitted.

4 Nordström M, Lindblad B, Anderson H, Bergquist D, Kjellström T. Deep venous thrombosis and occult malignancy: an epidemiological study. BMJ. 1994;308:891-4.

5 Sørensen HT, Mellemkjær L, Steffensen FH, Olsen JH, Nielsen GL. The risk of a diagnosis of cancer after primary deep venous thrombosis or pulmonary embolism. N Engl J Med. 1998;338:1169-73.

6 Baron JA, Gridley G, Weiderpass E, Nyrén O, Linet M. Venous thromboembolism and cancer. Lancet. 1998;351:1077-80.

Hæmostasis

Lectures

Haemostasis 2001;31(suppl. 1):43-44

Systemic Syndromes

Arterial thrombotic syndromes in cancer patients

BENJAMIN BRENNER
Thrombosis & Hemostasis Unit, Department of Hematology, Rambam Medical Center and Bruce Rappaport Faculty of Medicine, Technion, Haifa, Israel

A variety of arterial thrombotic syndromes can be observed in cancer patients. Most commonly involved sites are the peripheral arterial circulation of the lower or upper extremities, [1] and the cerebral vasculature [2]. The differential diagnosis of cerebral symptoms in cancer patients usually includes metastasis and hemorrhage.

Surprisingly there are no well-defined registries of arterial thrombosis in cancer patients. In the Stroke Register of the Hospital del Sagrat Cor in Barcelona, of 1,099 patients with first cerebrovascular episode, in one percent stroke was the form of onset of a previously unrecognized hematological malignancy [3]. Other unusual sites of arterial thrombosis in patients with cancer include the mesenteric renal and hepatic vessels.

A unique clinical entity in cancer patients is non-bacterial thrombotic endocarditis (NBTE), which can be observed in solid tumors and is particularly common in patients with myeloproliferative disorders. NBTE can complicate various malignancies and may cause morbidity and mortality mainly as a result of systemic embolism.

In a prospective echocardiographic screening of 200 nonselected ambulatory patients with solid tumors was performed [4]. Cardiac valvular vegetations were found in 38 patients (19%) compared with only 2/100 controls (2%, p< 0.001). Vegetations were found on the mitral or on the aortic valve in 19 and 18 patients, respectively.

Valvular lesions were mostly common in patients with carcinoma of the pancreas (3 of 6, 50%), carcinoma of the lung (9 of 32, 28%), and lymphoma (10 of 52, 19%).

Thromboembolism was diagnosed in 9 of 38 patients (24%) with vegetations compared with 13 of 162 patients without vegetations (8%; p=0.013).

In another study we have demonstrated echocardiographic valve abnormalities in 19 of 30 patients (63%) with myeloproliferative disorders [5].

Systemic arterial thrombotic syndromes in cancer patients include disseminated intra vascular coagulation (DIC) and thrombotic microangiopathy (TM) manifested as thrombotic thrombocytopenic purpura (TTP) or hemolytic uremic syndrome (HUS). This syndrome has been observed in many types of malignancies and is most commonly seen in gastric adenocarcinoma followed by carcinoma of the breast, colon and small cell carcinoma of the lung [6]. Chemotherapeutic drugs, which have been implicated in causing TM, include cisplatinum, 2-CDA and bleomycin. In addition, drugs that are used in supportive care for cancer patients including cyclosporine A, FK-506 and sulpha derivatives may also cause TM.

The incidence of TTP among 332 patients after unrelated allogeneic stem cell transplantation (SCT) was 6% compared to 2% of matched cell grafts [7]. The mortality rate was extremely high (86%) [7]. Of 131 leukemic children who underwent SCT 21% developed TTP at a median of 46 days. The risk was

KARGER

Fax +41 61 306 12 34
E-Mail karger@karger.ch
www.karger.com

0301-0147/00/0309/0001$17.50/0

Accessible online at:
www.karger.com/journals/hae

Benjamin Brenner
Rambam Medical Center - Thrombosis and Hemostasis Unit
Department of Hematology - P.O. Box 9602
Haifa 31096 - ISRAEL
Tel. +972/48342553 – 972/54521580 - Fax +972/48542343
b_brenner@rambam.health.gov.il

higher in patients receiving unrelated donor source of stem cells (p=0.020) [8].
Complete deficiency of von Willebrand factor-cleaving protease (VWF-cp) has recently been identified as a pathogenetically important factor for familial TTP. Partial deficiency of VWF-cp can be found in patients with neoplasia and TM [9]. Management of TTP/HUS in cancer patients is as in patients without cancer but the outcome particularly in patients with TTP after allogeneic transplant is grim despite intensive plasmapheresis. Role of alternative drugs like defibrotide remains to be established in this setting.
Potential pathogenetic mechanisms of arterial thrombosis in cancer patients may involve tumor cells interactions with coagulation factors, platelets and vessel wall. Laboratory findings may include enhanced platelet activation elevation of coagulation factor (VII and VIII) levels, a decrease in natural anticoagulants like protein C and protein S, APC-resistance and impaired fibrinolysis.
The potential devastating implications of arterial thrombosis necessitate antithrombotic modalities, which may include heparin, LMWH and vitamin K antagonists. The efficacy and safety of these agents have not been rigorously evaluated by prospective randomized trials. Likewise, the role, if any, of platelet antagonists in this setting has not been established.
Lack of data for these life-threatening syndromes suggests that prospective trials of arterial thrombosis in cancer patients are highly warranted.

References

1. Van Genderen PJ, Michiels JJ. Erythromelalgia: a pathogomonic microvascular thrombotic complication in essential thrombocythemia and polycythemia vera. Sem Thromb Hemost 1997;23:357-62.
2. Newton HB. Neurologic complications of systemic cancer. Am Fam Physician 1999;59:878-86.
3. Arboix A. Cerebrovascular disease in the cancer patient. Rev Neurol 2000;31:1250-2.
4. Edoute Y, Haim N, Rinkevich D, Brenner B, Reisner SA. Cardiac valvular vegetations in cancer patients: a prospective echocardiographic study of 200 patients. Am J Med 1997; 102:252-8.
5. Reisner SA, Rinkiewich D, Markiewicz W, Tatarsky I, Brenner B. Cardiac involvement in patients with myelo-proliferative disorders. Am J Med 1992;93:498-504.
6. Lessene JB, Rothschild N, Erickson B et al. Cancer-associated hemolytic-uremic syndrome: Analysis of 85 cases from a national registry. J Clin Oncol 1989;7:781-9.
7. Fuge R, Bird JM, Fraser A, Hart D, Hunt L, Comish JM, Goulden N, Oakhill A, Pamphilon DH, Steward CG, Marks DI. The clinical features, risk factors and outcome of thrombotic thrombocytopenic purpura occurring after bone marrow transplantation. Br J Haematol 2001; 113:58-64.
8. Uderzo C, Fumagalli M, De Lorenzo P, Busca A, Vassallo E, Bonanomi S, Lanino E, Dini G, Varotto S, Messina C, Miniero R, Valsecchi MG, Balduzzi A. Impact of thrombotic thrombocytopenic purpura on leukemic children undergoing bone marrow transplantation. Bone Marrow Transplant 2000;26:1005-9.
9. Fontana S, Gerritsen HE, Kremer Hovinga J, Furlan M, Lammle B. Microangiopathic haemolytic anaemia in metastasizing malignant tumours is not associated with a severe deficiency of the von Willebrand factor-cleaving protease. Br J Haematol 2001 113:100-2.

Hæmostasis

Lectures

Haemostasis 2001;31(suppl. 1):45-46

Autoimmune bleeding disorders in cancer patients

PIER MANNUCCIO MANNUCCI
Angelo Bianchi Bonomi Hemophilia and Thrombosis Center, IRCCS Maggiore Hospital and University of Milan, Italy

Introduction

Acquired hemophilia is an autoimmune disease resulting from the presence of autoantibodies directed against clotting factors. While this disorder may appear at any age, the elderly are most commonly affected. It is usually recognized by unprovoked hemorrhage into skin and muscles, or iatrogenic bleeding. In contrast, hemophilia is a congenital deficiency of either factor VIII or factor IX mainly associated with hemarthroses. Although persons with hemophilia may develop antibodies against factor VIII or factor IX, these are alloantibodies stimulated by exposure to exogenous factor concentrates.

Autoantibodies against all of the coagulation factors have been described, but those directed against factor VIII are the most common [1-4]. Recent advances in elucidating the structure-functional relationships of factor VIII have helped to identify "hot-spots" in the molecule which are the usual targets of the autoantibodies.

The incidence of acquired inhibitors of factor VIII has been estimated at 0.2-1.0 case per one million population per year [5] but many of the low titer antibodies may go unrecognized unless the affected individual is exposed to trauma or surgery. Bleeding manifestations are often dramatic, with 80-90% presenting with major hemorrhages and a 10-22% mortality rate directly or indirectly attributable to the inhibitor [4].

The age distribution of the autoantibodies is biphasic, with a small peak in young women post-partum, and the major peak in individuals of both sexes aged 60-80 years. The majority have been previously healthy, but in some there is a defined or evolving autoimmune or lymphoproliferative disorders. Associated immunologic disorders include systemic lupus erythematosus [6], rheumatoid arthritis [7] multiple sclerosis [8] and graft-versus-host disease after allogeneic bone marrow transplant [9]. Asthma, chronic inflammatory bowel disease, and pemphigus have also been reported [10]. Severe allergic reaction to antibiotics (penicillin and sulfonamides), alpha interferon [11] and BCG vaccination [12] are also associated with the development of autoantibodies to factor VIII.

In older persons malignant lymphoproliferative disorders such as chronic lymphoproliferative disorders, leukemia or lymphoma are commonly reported. In a retrospective analysis, Sallah et al [13] evaluated reports of acquired inhibitors and malignancy. They describe 41 patients, median age of 70, with solid tumors of the prostate and lung (25 patients), and leukemia or lymphoma. Bleeding manifestations included hematuria, gastrointestinal hemorrhage, and bleeding into soft tissues. Treatment of the underlying disorder with chemotherapy, surgery or hormonal manipulation led to the disappearance of the inhibitor in 22% of patients. The rest of the patients had disease that did not respond to treatment of either the tumor or the inhibitor. The authors postulate that inhibitors of coagulation may be a manifestation of a paraneoplastic syndrome.

The experience of our large hemophilia center is instructive. During a 20 years period, 80 patients with acquired hemophilia were seen at the haemophilia center. Their ages ranged from 20 to 99, but less than 10% were under 50. Associated diseases were found in 98 patients (41%), malignancy in 24%, rheumatological disease in 16% and postpartum in 11%.

The development of potent procoagulant concentrates has improved the management of bleeding and the unraveling of mechanisms of autoimmunity are currently suggesting new agents for immune modification that may be safer and more effective than the current immunosuppressive regimens.

KARGER

Fax +41 61 306 12 34
E-Mail karger@karger.ch
www.karger.com

0301-0147/00/0309/0001$17.50/0

Accessible online at:
www.karger.com/journals/hae

Pier Mannuccio Mannucci
Centro Emofilia e Trombosi - A. Bianchi Bonomi - Università di Milano
Via Pace, 9 - 20122 MILANO - ITALY
Tel. +39/02/5454425 - Fax. +39/02/5516093
piermannuccio.mannucci@unimi.it

References

1. Shapiro S and Hultin M. Acquired inhibitors to the blood coagulation factors. Sem Thromb Hemost 1975; 1: 336-385.
2. Lusher J, Hillman C. The effect of inhibitors on factor assays, in Advances in Coagulation Testing: Interpretation and Application, D. Tripplet, Editor. 1986 College of American Pathologists: Skokie, IL p. 73-83.
3. Palascak J. Autoantibodies against clotting factors, in Acquired Bleeding Disorders in Children: Abnormalities of Hemostasis, J. Lusher and M. Barnhart Editors. 1981, Masson Publishing Company: New York, p. 99-113.
4. Green D, Lechner K. A survey of 215 non-hemophilic patients with inhibitors to factor VIII. Thromb Haemost 1981. 45: 200-203.
5. Lottenberg R, Kenro T, Kitchesn C. Acquired haemophilia: a natural history of 16 patients with factor VIII inhibitors receiving little or no therapy. Arch Intern Med 1987; 147: 1077-1081.
6. Schulman S, et al. Cyclosporine therapy for acquired factor VIII inhibitor in a patient with systemic lupus erythematosus. Thromb Haemost 1996; 76: 344-346.
7. Deinocencio J, Lovell D, Gabriel C. Acquired factor VIII inhibitor in juvenile rheumatoid arthritis. Pediatrics 1994; 94: 550-553.
8. Hoyle C, Ludlam C. Acquired factor VIII inhibitor associated with multiple sclerosis successfully treated with porcine factor VIII Thromb Haemost 1987 ; 57 : 233.
9. Seidler C, et al. Spontaneous factor VIII inhibitor occurring in association with chronic graft-versus-host disease. Am J Hematol 1994; 24: 241-245.
10. Sohngen D, et al. Acquired factor VIII inhibitors in non hemophilic patients. Ann Hematol 1997; 74: 89-93.
11. Mauser-Bunschoten E, et al. Formation of antibodies to factor VIII in patients with hemophilia A who are treated with interferon for chronic hepatitis C. Ann Intern Med 1996; 125: 297-299.
12. Ferri G, et al. Development of factor VIII:C inhibitors following vaccination. Acta Haematologica 1996; 96: 110-111.
13. Sallah S, Wan J. Inhibitors against factor VIII in patients with cancer: analysis of 41 patients. Cancer 2001; 91: 1067-1074.

Hæmostasis

Lectures

Haemostasis 2001;31(suppl. 1):47-48

Cancer and DIC

MARCEL LEVI
Academic Medical Center, University of Amsterdam, the Netherlands

Introduction

Disseminated intravascular coagulation (DIC) is a syndrome that may complicate a variety of diseases, including malignant disease. DIC is characterized by a widespread and intravascular activation of coagulation (leading to intravascular fibrin deposition) and simultaneous consumption of coagulation factors and platelets (potentially resulting in bleeding) [1]. It is not clear to what extent the manifestation of clinically overt thrombo-embolism can be ascribed to malignancy-associated DIC. There is ample evidence for a procoagulant state in virtually all patients with advanced malignant disease, however, the incidence of overt DIC appears to be much lower [2].

The incidence of DIC in consecutive patients with solid tumors was found to be 7% in a recent clinical study [3] and in patients presenting with acute leukemia, in particular acute lymphoblastic leukemia, DIC can be diagnosed in 15-20% [4]. Some reports indicate that the incidence of DIC in acute leukemia patients might further increase during remission induction with chemotherapy [4]. In patients with acute promyelocytic leukemia (AML M-3) DIC may be diagnosed in more than 90% of patients at the time of diagnosis or after initiation of remission induction [5].

The coagulopathy that accompanies acute promyelocytic leukemia, is often seen as one of the most straightforward forms of DIC complicating malignancy [6].

However, this form of leukemia-associated hemostatic derangement can be considered as an exceptional type of DIC, characterized by a marked hyperfibrinolysis. The precise pathogenesis of this hyperfibrinolysis has not been elucidated.

A recent report points to a potential newly described receptor for fibrinolytic proteins, annexin II, that is expressed on the surface of leukemic cells in patients with acute promyelocytic leukemia. Annexin II may facilitate plasmin generation at the surface of the cells and may thereby play a pivotal role in the development of the hyperfibrinolytic state.

Despite the prominent role of hyperfibrinolysis in patients with acute promyelocytic leukemia, there is mounting evidence that this derangement is superimposed on a more common presentation of DIC, characterized by coagulation activation and fibrin deposition. Indeed, diffuse thrombosis is found in 15-25% of cases at autopsy and recent studied have demonstrated tissue-factor dependent activation of coagulation in this patient category.

Solid tumor cells can express different procoagulant molecules including tissue factor (TF), which assembles with factor VII(a) to activate factors IX and X, and a cancer procoagulant (CP), a cysteine protease with factor X activating properties [7]. Recent studies show the occurrence of TF in vascular endothelial cells as well as tumor cells in breast cancer, while not appearing in material from patients with benign fibrocystic breast disease, while TF was functionally active [8]. It should be noted that the roles of TF in pathophysiology are only partly understood as yet. Independent from its clotting cofactor function TF appears to be involved in tumor metastasis [9] and angiogenesis [10], factors that may di-rectly influence the course of malignancy and affect the occurrence of thrombosis.

Clinically, DIC in cancer has in general a less fulminant presentation than the types of DIC complicating sepsis and trauma.

A more gradual, but also more chronic, systemic activation of coagulation can proceed subclinically. Eventually this process may lead to exhaustion of platelets and coagulation factors and bleeding (for example at the site of the tumor) may be the first clinical symptom indicating the presence of DIC. If the function of the liver is not compromised, enhanced synthesis of coagulation proteins may mask the ongoing consumption of factors and in that case thrombocytopenia is the most prominent sign of ongoing DIC.

KARGER
Fax +41 61 306 12 34
E-Mail karger@karger.ch
www.karger.com

0301-0147/00/0309/0001$17.50/0

Accessible online at:
www.karger.com/journals/hae

Marcel Levi
Academic Medical Center - Department of Internal Medicine
University of Amsterdam - Meibergdreef 9
Amsterdam AZ 1105 - THE NETHERLANDS
Tel. +31/20/5662171 - Fax +31/20/6919658
m.m.levi@amc.uva.nl

Measurement of fibrin-related markers (such as soluble fibrin or fibrin degradation products) may be helpful in establishing the diagnosis in a routine setting, however, the specificity of these tests in cancer-related DIC has not been established so far. The therapeutic cornerstone of DIC is treatment of the underlying disorder. In fact, if the malignant disease can be brought in remission, the DIC will simultaneously disappear.
Supportive therapy may consist of anticoagulant treatment, however, the efficacy and safety of this strategy in cancer patients with DIC has never been studied in sound clinical studies. The administration of platelets, plasma or plasma derivatives is only useful in case of bleeding or if there is a high risk of bleeding.
The role of restoring defective physiological anticoagulant pathways (e.g. by administration of antithrombin or activated protein C concentrates) has never been evaluated.

References

1. Levi M, ten Cate H. Disseminated intravascular coagulation. N Engl J Med 1999;341:586-592.
2. Colman RW, Rubin RN. Disseminated intravascular coagulation due to malignancy. Seminars in Oncology 1990;17:172-186.
3. Sallah S, Wan JY, Nguyen NP, Hanrahan LR, Sigounas G. Disseminated intravascular coagulation in solid tumors: clinical and pathological study. Thromb.Haemost. 2001;86:828-833.
4. Sarris AH, Kempin S, Berman E, Michaeli J, Little C, Andreeff M, et al. High incidence of disseminated intravascular coagulation during remission induction of adult patients with acute lymphoblastic leukemia. Blood 1992;79:1305-1310.
5. Avvisati G, ten Cate JW, Sturk A, Lamping R, Petti MG, Mandelli F. Acquired alpha-2-antiplasmin deficiency in acute promyelocytic leukaemia. Br.J Haematol. 1988;70:43-48.
6. Tallman MS. The thrombophilic state in acute promyelocytic leukemia. Semin.Thromb.Hemost. 1999;25:209-215.
7. Donati MB. Cancer and thrombosis: from Phlegmasia alba dolens to transgenic mice. Thromb.Haemost. 1995;74:278-281.
8. Contrino J, Hair G, Kreutzer DL, Rickles FR. In situ detection of tissue factor in vascular endothelial cells: correlation with the malignant phenotype of human breast disease. Nature Medicine 1996;2:209-215.
9. Bromberg ME, Konigsberg WH, Madison JF, Pawashe A, Garen A. Tissue factor promotes melanoma metastasis by a pathway independent of blood coagulation. Proc. Natl. Acad. Sci. U.S.A. 1995;92:8205-8209.
10. Zhang Y, Deng Y, Luther T, Muller M, Ziegler R, Waldherr R, et al. Tissue factor controls the balance of angiogenic and antiangiogenic properties of tumor cells in mice. J Clin. Invest. 1994;94:1320-1327.

Hæmostasis

Lectures

Haemostasis 2001;31(suppl. 1):49-51

The coagulopathy of acute promyelocytic leukemia

FRANCESCO RODEGHIERO
Hematology Department, San Bortolo Hospital, Vicenza, Italy

Acute promyelocytic leukemia (APL) accounts for about 10-15% of acute myeloid leukemias in adults. Two forms have been described: the common hypergranular type associated with leukopenia and the more rare (25% of cases), more aggressive form associated with hyperleukocytosis and scarcely granulated blasts, described as microgranular variant. Both types are invariably characterized by the balanced reciprocal translocation t(15;17) which fuses the PML gene on chromosome 15 to the retinoic acid receptor a (RAR-α) gene on chromosome 17, generating the PML/RAR-α chimeric gene. The PML/RAR-α protein acts in a dominant negative manner, as an aberrant retinoid receptor with altered DNA-binding and transcriptional regulatory properties, and inhibits the cellular signalling by physiological concentration of all-trans retinoic acid (ATRA).

A peculiar coagulopathy with several clotting abnormalities and hemorrhagic symptoms is almost invariably associated to APL and is worsened by chemotherapy [1,2]. Life-threatening hemorrhages may occur at presentation or more frequently during the first days of treatment, with a reported incidence of early hemorrhagic deaths of 10-20 % [2,3]. The pathophysiology, clinical relevance and treatment of the APL associated coagulopathy will be briefly addressed.

Pathophysiology of APL coagulopathy

Abnormalities of the laboratory coagulation tests showing reduction of fibrinogen and increased fibrin degradation products, with variably prolonged coagulation tests, are compatible with a diagnosis of disseminated intravascular coagulation (DIC). However, platelet count is reduced due to both intravascular consumption and bone marrow failure, hence thrombocytopenia cannot be used as an adjunctive criterium for DIC diagnosis. In addition, the contribution to the coagulopathy of other mechanisms including fibrinolysis and proteolysis cannot be overlooked. Indeed leukemic promyelocytes contain procoagulant (tissue factor (TF), cancer procoagulant (CP)), fibrinolytic (urokinase-type plasminogen activator, u-PA; tissue-type plasminogen activator, t-PA) and proteolytic (elastase, chymotrypsin) substances that could be expressed on their surface or released into the bloodstream. Recent sensitive immunological methods able to detect enzyme-inhibitor complexes and trace amount of activation peptides of the coagulation / fibrinolysis / proteolysis pathways have demonstrated that all these systems are involved. However, the key event is represented by thrombin intravascular generation as shown by the constant increase of D-dimer, a specific lysis product of cross-linked fibrin, which definitively shows that hyperfibrinolysis, rarely an overwhelming phenomenon, invariably occurs as a secondary event [4]. None of several parameters investigated, apart, possibly, from fibrinogen level and platelet count seems to be a reliable risk factor of bleeding [2].

Clinical relevance and treatment of the APL coagulopathy

Before ATRA availability, several anecdotal studies provided inconsistent evidence on the effectiveness of treating clotting abnormalities with heparin, in order to quench the intravascular clotting or antifibrinolytics to control the hyperfibrinolysis. As shown by a retrospective study involving 268 consecutive patients, the high rate of early hemorrhagic deaths was not reduced by the use of heparin and/or antifibrinolytics in comparison to supportive therapy alone, even in recent years when platelet transfusions became widely available [3].

The introduction of ATRA, which is able to restore the RAR-α dependent cellular signaling and to induce differentiation and apoptosis of APL blast cells, together with anthracycline based chemotherapy, has

KARGER

Fax +41 61 306 12 34
E-Mail karger@karger.ch
www.karger.com

0301-0147/00/0309/0001$17.50/0

Accessible online at:
www.karger.com/journals/hae

Francesco Rodeghiero
Divisione di Ematologia - U.L.SS. n. 6
Via Rodolfi, 37 - 36100 VICENZA - ITALY
Tel. +39/0444/993626 - Fax +39/0444/920708
rodeghiero@hemato.ven.it

dramatically improved the overall survival of APL patients with a cure rate up to 75%. In addition, since from early pilot studies with ATRA, clinicians observed that the rapid resolution of the bleeding symptoms and the higher remission rates obtained appeared mainly associated with a substantial reduction of early hemorrhagic deaths and resistant cases (usually less than 10%). A number of experimental and observational studies, carefully reviewed by the Bergamo group [4], have shown that ATRA dramatically influences the hemostatic system including the endothelial department. Indeed ATRA decreases the expression of TF and CP without affecting the global fibrinolytic activities of APL blasts and is able to counteract the thrombogenic stimuli on endothelium by opposing to both the thrombomodulin downregulation and the TF upregulation exerted by the increased level of TNF-α and IL-1β [5].

However, despite the rapid amelioration of coagulation abnormalities, no significant difference in the incidence of early hemorrhagic death (still around 5%) was observed on the basis of the only two randomised studies evaluating the impact of ATRA alone vs. chemotherapy alone in induction. Furthermore, in a study comparing ATRA and idarubicin (499 cases) vs. idarubicin alone (123 cases) in two historic series of patients treated by the same Italian cooperative group [6], the rate of early (within 10 days from treatment) hemorrhagic deaths was 2.4 and 4.1 % respectively, showing a favourable trend for ATRA patients but not reaching statistical significance, a finding confirmed also by a recent study [7]. Thus, although there is a common consensus that ATRA ameliorates the APL coagulopathy, the real contribution in the reduction of hemorrhagic deaths remains doubtful and its major impact is evident in terms of complete remission and overall survival.

In the light of the complex effect of ATRA, the lack of evidence of clinical benefit and the report of arterial thrombosis in APL, active hemostatic agents including antifibrinolitics should be generally avoided in these patients, whereas substitutive treatment with fresh frozen plasma and platelet remains fundamental.

Future studies will show the contribution of arsenic trioxide and other arsenic compounds towards a better treatment in this leukaemia, already cured in a high proportion of cases.

These agents are active in inducing apoptosis and differentiation in APL blasts resistant to ATRA, and induce hemostatic changes similar to those observed with ATRA [8]. It might be well that these agent could contribute to APL cure in a more complex way than previously thought in which the interweaving effects on the leukemic cells, the endothelium and the hemostatic system play a major role, as suggested by a recent study showing inhibition of increased angiogenesis by ATRA in APL [9].

References

1. Warrel RP: Pathogenesis and management of acute promyelocytic leukemia. Ann Rev Med 1996; 47: 555.
2. Rodeghiero F, Castaman G: The pathophysiology and treatment of hemorrhagic syndrome of acute promylocytic leukemia. Leukemia 1994; 8, suppl 2, 20-26.
3. Rodeghiero F, Avvisati G, Castaman G, Barbui T, Mandelli F:Early deaths and anti-hemorrhagic treatments in acute promyelocytic leukemia. A GIMEMA retrospective study in 268 consecutive patients. Blood 1990; 75, 2112-2117.
4. Barbui T, Finazzi G, Falanga A: The impact of All-trans retinoic acid on the coagulopathy of acute promyelocytic leukemia. Blood, 1998, 3093-3101.
5. Falanga A, Marchetti M, Giovanelli S, Barbui T: All-trans- retinoic acid counteracts endothelial cell procoagulant activity induced by a human promyelocytic leukemia-derived cell line (NB4). Blood 1996; 87, 613.
6. Di Bona E, Avvisati G, Castaman G, Vegna M L, De Sanctis V, Rodeghiero F, Mandelli F: Early haemorrhagic morbidity and mortality during remission induction with o without all-trans retinoic acid in acute promyelocytic leukaemia. Br J Haematol 2000, 108, 689-695.
7. Burnett A K, Grimwade D, Solomon E, Wheathley K, Goldstone A H: Presenting white blood cell count and kinetics of molecular remission predict prognosis in acute promyelocytic leukemia treated with All-trans retinoic acid: result of the randomized MRC trial. Blood 1999; 93, 4131-4143.
8. Chen Z, Chen G, Shen Z, Chen S, Wang Z: Treatment of acute promyelocytic leukemia with aarsenic compounds: in vivo and in vitro studies. Sem Hematol 2001; 38, 26-36.
9. Kini A R, Peterson, L C, Tallman M S, Lingen M W: Angiogenesis in acute promyelocytic leukemia: induction by vascular endothelial growth factor and inhibition by all-trans retinoic acid. Blood 2001; 97, 3919-3924.

Hæmostasis

Lectures

Haemostasis 2001;31(suppl. 1):52-54

Platelets, fibrinolysis and cancer

Cancer metastasis: a model of cell-protease and cell-cell interactions

MARIA BENEDETTA DONATI

Department of Vascular Medicine and Pharmacology, Istituto di Ricerche Farmacologiche Mario Negri, Consorzio Mario Negri Sud, Santa Maria Imbaro, Italy.

Cancer cells contribute to metastasis formation in distant organs by a complex machinery which involves both cell-cell crosstalks and the availability of cell proteases [1, 2].

Cell-cell interactions: Cancer cells may directly activate blood platelets, may come in contact with endothelial cells in the process of adhesion and migration through the vessel wall and may be supported by granulocytes in their interaction with endothelial cells [3]. Moreover, tumor-associated macrophages are stimulated by the cancer "milieu" to express cytokines, as well as procoagulant and fibrinolytic enzymes which can further influence the invasive capacity of tumor cells themselves [4, 5]. On the other hand, out of the many lytic enzymes proposed to play a role in tumor metastatic ability, collagenase and other metalloproteases, but particularly the plasminogen activator urokinase appears to be closely related to the adhesion machinery of tumor cells.

Urokinase/integrin interactions: Recent evidence indicates that migratory cells use both adhesion receptors and proteolytic enzymes to regulate their interaction with and response to extracellular matrices. This protease crosstalk occurs with integrins at several levels: integrin signalling induces proteases, proteases co-localyze with integrins and proteases regulate the interface between integrins and the intracellular cytoskeleton.

The urokinase/ urokinase receptor (u-PAR) /plasmin system is particularly of interest in this context. Urokinase, indeed, promotes the binding of its receptor (u-PAR) to a set of ß1 and ß2 integrins, which become activated, thus leading to promotion of cell migration [6, 7]. It has recently been demonstrated that u-PA binding to its receptor stimulates tumor cell migration by enhancing integrin-mediated signal transduction [8].

For integrin signalling the activation of src-family kinases would be particularly important [9]. It has even been proposed that u-PAR, ß2-integrins, src-kinases would form a single receptor complex in human monocytes and other migratory cells. The in vivo role of such interaction is supported by evidence that u-PAR and integrins cooperate to favour migration in vivo and that leukocytes recruitment is impaired in u-PAR deficient mice [10, 11].

Integrins: The role of cellular integrins in the control of metastatic potential, on the other hand, has been supported by many biological and pharmacological data with inhibitors or antibodies directed agonist αIIbß3 receptors expressed not only by platelets but also by different types of tumor cells [12]. In many studies the expression of these integrins correlated with the platelet aggregating ability and with the degree of invasiveness of the same cells and of tumor progression. More particularly, the degree of integrin activation appears important in this context, as shown by experiments where only breast cancer cells (isolated from human metastasis) which had αVß3 in the activated state were able to arrest on platelets, during blood flow in vitro, and promoted metatasis in a mouse model in vivo [13]. These observations strenghten the hypothesis that alterations in the control of integrin (particularly ß3)

KARGER

Fax +41 61 306 12 34
E-Mail karger@karger.ch
www.karger.com

0301-0147/00/0309/0001$17.50/0

Accessible online at:
www.karger.com/journals/hae

Maria Benedetta Donati
Consorzio Mario Negri Sud - Centro di Ricerche Biomediche e Farmacologiche
Via Nazionale, 1 - 66030 S. MARIA IMBARO (CH) - ITALY
Tel. +39/0872/570311 - Fax +39/0872/570299
donati@cmns.mnegri.it

activation within tumor cells, may influence their metastatic potential.

Selectins: Selectins (particularly P-selectin from blood platelets and endothelial cells and E-selectin from endothelial cells) are a class of adhesion molecules whose role has been clearly recognized in the multistep process leading to entry of circulating leukocytes into tissues during inflammation. In this context, selectins have shown to mediate attachment and rolling of circulating leukocytes which are finally arrested on the vessel wall with the cooperation of activated integrins. Our group has recently proposed an integrated model of P-selectin, its receptor P-selectin glycoprotein ligand-1 (PSGL-1) and ß-3 integrins with the intermediate step of intracellular tyrosine phosphorylation events, to give a biochemical basis to the process of PMN arrest on the vascular wall with the cooperation of blood platelets [14, 15]. It now appears increasingly clear that, during the process of metastatization, tumor cells recapitulate the adhesion cascade used by normal circulating cells (such as platelets or leukocytes) to interact with endothelial cells and start the process of extravation. The Figure outlines schematically the recruitment of tumor cells at sites of vascular damage.
In particular, the role of P-selectin in platelet tumor cell-adhesion has been repeatedly underlined both with in vitro and in vivo experiments; the latter include the observation that, in P-selectin knock-out mice, human colon carcinoma cells grow at lower rate and form a reduced number of tumor cell/platelet clumps in the lung vasculature [16]. Different P-selectin receptors have been identified in different tumor cell lines thus opening the way of rather selective interventions in order to block with new tools cell/cell interactions relevant for metastasis formation [12].

In conclusion, interactions of different normal cells with tumor cells, involving adhesion molecules and proteases, may be studied in relation to tumor cell metastatic potential and its possible control.

TUMOR CELL/PLATELET/VASCULAR WALL INTERACTIONS RECAPITULATE LEUKOCYTE RESPONSES IN INFLAMMATION.

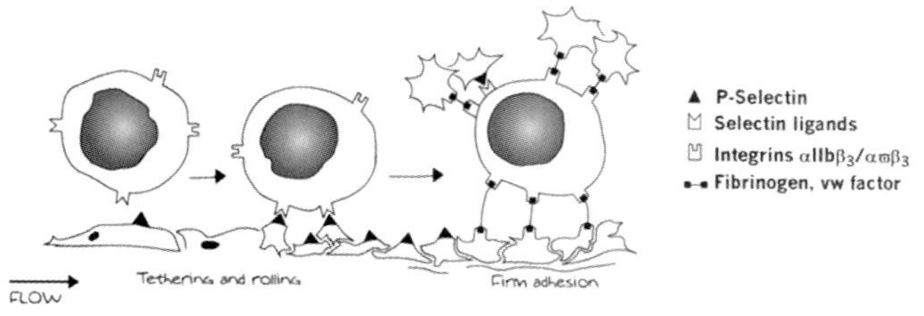

Platelets activated at a site of vascular damage mediate tumor cell recruitment through P-selectin-dependent tethering and rolling and β3 integrin-dependent firm adhesion.

References

1. Donati MB: Cancer and thrombosis: from Phlegmasia alba dolens to transgenic mice. Thromb Haemost 1995;74:278-281.
2. Poggi A, Rossi C, Beviglia L, Calabrese R, Donati MB: Platelets-tumor cell interactions; in Joseph M (ed): The Handbook of Immuno-pharmacology - Immuno-pharmacology of platelets. London, Academic Press, 1995, pp. 151-165.
3. Falanga A., Donati M.B. Pathogenesis of thrombosis in patients with malignancy. Int. J. Hematol., 2001; 73: 137-144.
4. Mussoni L, Donati MB: Expression of plasminogen activator as a marker of stimulation in tumor-associated macrophages. Haemostasis 1988;18:66-71.
5. Semeraro N, Colucci M: Tissue Factor in health and disease. Thromb Haemost 1997;78:759-764.
6. Chapman HA, Wei Y. Protease crosstalk with integrins: the urokinase receptor paradigm. Thromb Haemost. 2001; 86(1):124-9.
7. Simon DI, Wei Y, Zhang L, Rao NK, Xu H, Chen Z, Liu Q, Rosenberg S, Chapman HA. Identification of a urokinase receptor-integrin interaction site. Promiscuous regulator of integrin function. J Biol Chem. 2000; 275(14):10228-34.
8. Yebra M, Goretzki L, Pfeifer M, Mueller BM. Urokinase-type plasminogen activator binding to its receptor stimulates tumor cell migration by enhancing integrin-mediated signal transduction. Exp Cell Res. 1999; 250(1):231-40.
9. Degryse B, Resnati M, Rabbani SA, Villa A, Fazioli F, Blasi F. Src-dependence and pertussis-toxin sensitivity of urokinase receptor-dependent chemotaxis and cytoskeleton reorganization in rat smooth muscle cells. Blood; 1999; 94(2):649-6.
10. Gyetko MR, Sud S, Kendall T, Fuller JA, Newstead MW, Standiford TJ. Urokinase receptor-deficient mice have impaired neutrophil recruitment in response to pulmonary Pseudomonas aeruginosa infection. J Immunol.; 2000; 165(3):1513-9.
11. May AE, Kanse SM, Lund LR, Gisler RH, Imhof BA, Preissner KT. Urokinase receptor (CD87) regulates leukocyte recruitment via beta 2 integrins in vivo. J Exp Med. 1998; 188(6):1029-37.
12. Donati M.B., Evangelista V. Platelets and tumors. IN: Platelets in thrombotic and non thrombotic disorders, Gresele P., Page C., Vermylen J., Fuster V. Cambridge University Press, in press
13. Felding-Habermann B, O'Toole TE, Smith JW, Fransvea E, Ruggeri ZM, Ginsberg MH, Hughes PE, Pampori N, Shattil SJ, Saven A, Mueller BM. Integrin activation controls metastasis in human breast cancer. Proc Natl Acad Sci U S A 2001; 98: 1853-1858.
14. Cerletti C., Evangelista V., de Gaetano G. P-selectin-ß2 integrin cross-talk: a molecular mechanism for polymorpho-nuclear leukocyte recruitment at the site of vascular damage. Thromb. Haemost.; 1999, 82: 787-793.
15. Piccardoni P., Sideri R., Manarini S., Piccoli A., Martellli N., de Gaetano G., Cerletti C., Evangelista V. Platelet/polymorphonuclear leukocytes adhesion: a new role for src kinases in MAC-1 adhesive function triggered by P-selectin. Blood; 2001, 98: 108-116.
16. Kim YJ, Borsig L, Varki NM, Varki A. P-selectin deficiency attenuates tumor growth and metastasis. Proc Natl Acad Sci U S A 1998; 95: 9325-9330.

Hæmostasis

Lectures

Haemostasis 2001;31(suppl. 1):55-58

Tumor cell–platelet interaction in metastatic disease

BRUNHILDE FELDING-HABERMANN
The Scripps Research Institute, La Jolla, CA, USA

Metastasis of solid tumors to major target organs often involves tumor cell dissemination via the blood stream. Clinical and experimental evidence suggests that platelets may play a role in this process. Cancer is often associated with a high incidence of thrombosis [1]. The most severe forms are disseminated intravascular coagulation, migratory thrombophlebitis and pulmonary embolism. But even in the absence of clinically detected thromboembolic events, coagulation parameters are frequently elevated in cancer patients, and platelet turnover is generally enhanced. A combination of anticoagulant medication with established anti-cancer regimens resulted in improved therapeutic effects in a variety of malignancies.

Dissemination of metastasizing cells within the blood stream is thought to be supported by an interaction between tumor cells and platelets [2]. Perhaps the most convincing evidence is that experimental thrombocytopenia reduced hematogenous tumor metastasis in animal models. This effect was reversed upon platelet infusion [3]. Furthermore, inhibition of specific platelet adhesive functions by monoclonal antibodies, or synthetic and naturally occurring RGD-containing peptides reduced experimental metastasis significantly in the majority of studies. Metastasis was inhibited regardless of the tumor cell ability to induce platelet aggregation. Two mechanisms of platelet involvement in tumor metastasis can be distinguished: first, the induction of platelet activation and platelet aggregation by tumor cells or their released factors, which may be accompanied by passive entrapment of tumor cells into platelet aggregates; and second, a specific adhesive interaction between platelets and tumor cells. Both of these mechanisms are influenced by blood flow and flow dependent shear forces that are present in the vasculature. Under these conditions, an interaction between tumor cells and platelets may facilitate metastatic dissemination in at least three major ways: First, heteroaggregate formation could support tumor cell arrest within the blood stream, as a prerequisite for tumor cell extravasation; Second, association of tumor cells with platelets may reduce tumor cell exposure to mechanical stress and shear forces, which have been hypothesized to be a main cause of rapid cancer cell death in the vasculature: Third, tumor cells surrounded by platelets could be protected against immune defense mechanisms. In a platelet rich microenvironment, the tumor cells are exposed to platelet released factors that can promote tumor cell survival and proliferation, even at the site of arrest within blood vessels [4]. Platelet derived particles can further induce or intensify tumor cell invasive activity [5].

Comparative experimental data justify the concept that cancer cell attachment inside blood vessels is not merely due to passive entrapment of the tumor cells based on their diameter, but that it rather depends on active and specific interactions between tumor cells and the endothelium, or exposed sites of the subendothelial matrix. Most tumor cells express a variety of adhesion receptors, which may support their attachment to counter receptors or ligands at the endothelium, and to components of the subendothelial matrix. These include von Willebrand Factor, collagen, fibronectin, laminin, vitronectin and glycosaminoglycans. Specific adhesion of various tumor cell types to each of these matrix components has been demonstrated under static conditions. Adhesion receptors involved include members of the integrin family, as well as non-integrin receptors. Static conditions, however, are unlikely to occur in the circulation. Passive entrapment of tumor cells in narrow capillary vessels may temporarily interrupt blood flow and favor direct tumor cell attachment to the endothelium, or to exposed sites of the subendothelial matrix. However, shear rates can also reach maximal levels in capillary passages. Therefore,

KARGER
Fax +41 61 306 12 34
E-Mail karger@karger.ch
www.karger.com

0301-0147/00/0309/0001$17.50/0

Accessible online at:
www.karger.com/journals/hae

Brunilde Felding-Habermann
The Scripps Research Institute, MEM 175 - 10550 North Torrey Pines Road
La Jolla, CA 92037
Tel. +1/858/7842021 - Fax +1/858/7842030
brunie@scripps.edu

adhesion mechanisms that mediate tumor cell attachment to the vessel wall have to be designed such that an adhesive interaction can establish under flow conditions and continuously withstand shear stress. Tumor cell interaction with platelets may provide the tumor cells with specific mechanisms that physiologically mediate platelet anchorage during blood flow. Recent experimental evidence supports this concept. Adhesion receptors of the selectin and integrin families with their ligands, were reported to promote tumor cell-platelet interaction during blood flow and promote metastasis from the blood stream. Platelet P-selectin was shown to bind tumor cell sialyl Lewis$^{x/a}$ glycoprotein, and this mechanism promoted arrest of tumor cell-platelet emboli in the vasculature of target organs [6]. Tumor cell arrest was inhibited by heparin, based on its ability to interfere with P-selectin mediated platelet-tumor cell binding, rather than on heparins anticoagulant effect [7].

We recently identified a specific mechanism for tumor cell-platelet interaction during blood flow. This mechanism is based on binding of platelet integrin $\alpha IIb\beta 3$ to tumor cell integrin $\alpha v\beta 3$ via divalent crosslinking ligands [8]. This was documented for human melanoma cells and fibrinogen as a possible ligand bridge. The interaction of tumor cells and platelets lead to tumor cell arrest and depended on platelet adhesive functions. The same mechanism supported human breast cancer cell arrest during blood flow in an established breast cancer cell model, and in freshly isolated metastatic cells from peripheral blood samples and malignant effusions of stage IV breast cancer patients [9] (Fig. 1). Importantly, the platelet interactive phenotype in breast cancer cells was associated with the metastatic phenotype. Metastasis derived variants of the breast cancer cell line, but not the parental cells themselves, were able to utilize integrin $\alpha v\beta 3$ for platelet binding and for arrest during blood flow. The parental tumor cells and their metastatic variants expressed $\alpha v\beta 3$ at the same levels. Therefore, integrin $\alpha v\beta 3$ can exist in breast cancer cells in an activated and a non-activated functional state. The expression of activated, platelet interactive $\alpha v\beta 3$ is associated with the metastatic phenotype. This was confirmed by introducing a constitutively activated mutant $\alpha 3$ subunit into a $\alpha 3$-negative variant of the parental breast cancer cells, which resulted in a platelet interactive and highly metastatic tumor cell phenotype (Fig. 1). Thus, alterations within tumors that lead to the aberrant control of integrin activation are expected to adversely affect the course of human breast cancer.

In order to clarify definitively, whether platelets indeed play a critical role in tumor metastasis, we are now establishing a new mouse model that lacks circulating platelets, and that is immune deficient to accept human tumor cell grafts. This model is based on a defect in the p45 subunit of the hematopoietic transcription factor NF-E2, which is required for platelet maturation [10]. We established the NF-E2 mutant allele on a scid/scid genetic background, and this model will allow us to analyze the metastatic activity of human tumor cells in the absence or presence of circulating platelets.

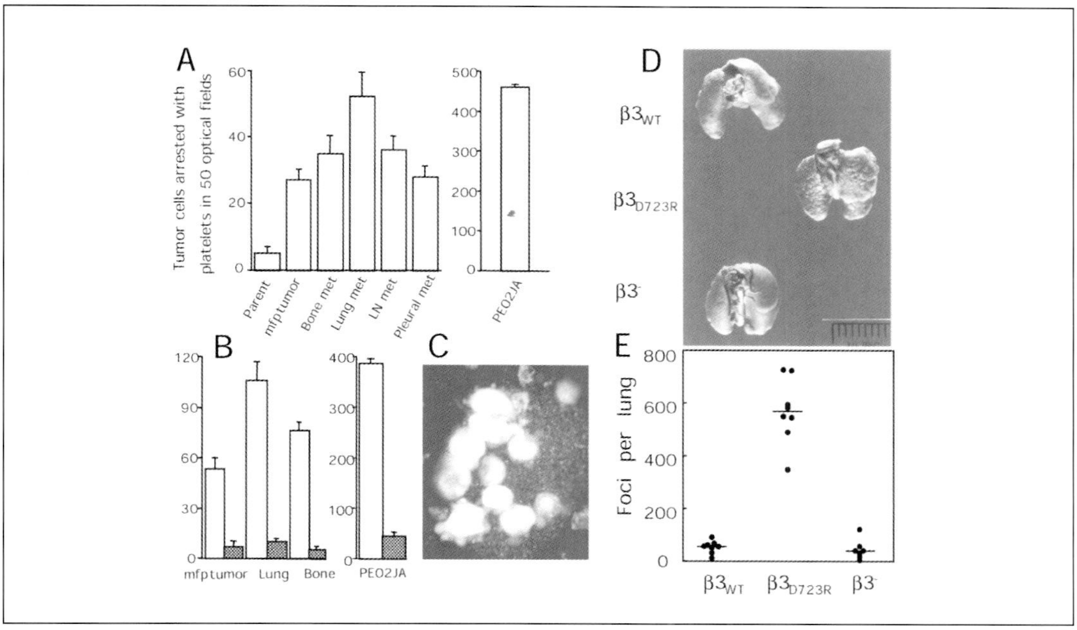

Figure 1. *Expression of activated integrin αvβ3 in human breast cancer cells promotes platelet-mediated tumor cell arrest during blood flow and experimental metastasis.*
A. *MDA-MB 435 cell variants derived from mammary fat pad (mfp) tumors or metastases (bone, lung, lymph node or the pleural cavity) in SCID mice, but not the parental cell population at large, bind to activated platelets and utilize this mechanism for cell arrest during blood flow. Tumor cells were stained with hydroethidine (red fluorescence), suspended in normal donor blood containing mepacrine (green fluorescence) and 50 nM H-D-Phe-Pro-Arg-chloromethyl ketone hydrochloride as anticoagulant. This suspension was perfused over a thrombogenic collagen I matrix at a venous wall shear rate of 50 sec*$^{-1}$ *(4 dynes/cm*^{2}*) [8]. Under these conditions, platelets attach to the matrix, become activated and form thrombi. During perfusion, tumor cell interaction with thrombi was monitored by video microscopy and image acquisition at predefined positions with filter settings that discern platelet specific and tumor cell specific fluorescent signal. Thrombus formation at the matrix and a negligible number of directly attached tumor cells (not shown) were unaffected by the tumor cell type. The right panel shows primary metastatic tumor cells isolated from a pleural effusion of a patient with stage IV breast cancer (PE02JA) analyzed under the same conditions. The y-axes in A and B denote the number of tumor cells that arrested through association with platelets.* ***B.*** *Breast cancer cell interaction with platelets depends on tumor cell integrin αvβ3 and platelet integrin αIIbβ3 function. Mammary fat pad (mfp) tumor or metastasis (lung, bone) derived variants of MDA-MB 435 cells were analyzed as above in the absence (open bars) or presence (hatched bars) of 80 μg/ml function blocking anti αvβ3 mab VNR1 27.1. This antibody inhibits tumor cell platelet interaction, but not thrombus formation. Anti-αIIbβ3 mab LJ-CP8 inhibits thrombus formation and abolishes tumor cell binding (not shown). Note that all tested MDA-MB 435 cell variants express equivalent levels of αvβ3, but no platelet integrin αIIbβ3 (not shown).* ***C.*** *Projection of confocal sections through a breast cancer cell containing thrombus, acquired during blood perfusion. These tumor cells (PE02JA) were freshly isolated from a pleural effusion of a patient with advanced breast cancer and displayed a highly platelet interactive phenotype (right panel in A).* ***D.*** *Activation of integrin αvβ3 promotes metastasis in MDA-MB 435 human breast cancer cells. Comparison of in vitro generated variants of MDA-MB 435 cells that either lack α3 integrin expression (α3 minus) or were transfected to express αvβ3 wild type (*$\alpha 3_{WT}$*) or constitutively activated mutant avb3* $_{D723R}$ *(*$\alpha 3_{D723R}$*). The cell variants (1x10*^{6}*) were injected into the lateral tail veins of 8-week old female C.B-17 scid/scid mice, and metastatic foci analyzed at the surface of the lungs after 42 days. Representative lungs are shown. E. Numbers of foci per lung (group size n=8). Cells expressing activated* $\alpha v\beta 3_{D723R}$ *produced significantly more metastases than cells lacking α3 or expressing non-activated αvβ3* $_{WT}$ *(*$p < 0.0001$ *by the Kruskal Wallis test).*

References

1. Rickles, F. R. and Levine, M. N. Epidemiology of thrombosis in cancer. Acta Haematol., 106: 6-12, 2001.
2. Nierodzik, M. L., Klepfish, A., and Karpatkin, S. Role of platelets, thrombin, integrin IIb-IIIa, fibronectin and von Willebrand factor on tumor adhesion in vitro and metastasis in vivo. Thromb.Haemost., 74: 282-290, 1995.
3. Gasic, G. J. Role of plasma, platelets, and endothelial cells in tumor metastasis. Cancer Metastasis Rev., 3: 99-114, 1984.
4. Al Mehdi, A. B., Tozawa, K., Fisher, A. B., Shientag, L., Lee, A., and Muschel, R. J. Intravascular origin of metastasis from the proliferation of endothelium-attached tumor cells: a new model for metastasis. Nat.Med., 6: 100-102, 2000.
5. Lindenmeyer, F., Legrand, Y., and Menashi, S. Upregulation of MMP-9 expression in MDA-MB231 tumor cells by platelet granular membrane. FEBS Lett., 418: 19-22, 1997.
6. Kim, Y. J., Borsig, L., Varki, N. M., and Varki, A. P-selectin deficiency attenuates tumor growth and metastasis. Proc.Natl.Acad.Sci.U.S.A., 95: 9325-9330, 1998.
7. Borsig, L., Wong, R., Feramisco, J., Nadeau, D. R., Varki, N. M., and Varki, A. Heparin and cancer revisited: Mechanistic connections involving platelets, P-selectin, carcinoma mucins, and tumor metastasis. Proc.Natl.Acad.Sci.U.S.A, 98: 3352-3357, 2001.
8. Felding-Habermann, B., Habermann, R., Saldivar, E., and Ruggeri, Z. M. Role of beta3 integrins in melanoma cell adhesion to activated platelets under flow. J.Biol.Chem., 271: 5892-5900, 1996.
9. Felding-Habermann, B., O'Toole, T. E., Smith, J. W., Fransvea, E., Ruggeri, Z. M., Ginsberg, M. H., Hughes, P. E., Pampori, N., Shattil, S. J., Saven, A., and Mueller, B. M. Integrin activation controls metastasis in human breast cancer. Proc.Natl.Acad.Sci.U.S.A, 98: 1853-1858, 2001.
10. Shivdasani, R. A., Rosenblatt, M. F., Zucker-Franklin, D., Jackson, C. W., Hunt, P., Saris, C. J., and Orkin, S. H. Transcription factor NF-E2 is required for platelet formation independent of the actions of thrombopoietin/MGDF in megakaryocyte development. Cell, 81: 695-704, 1995.

Hæmostasis

Lectures

Haemostasis 2001;31(suppl. 1):59

u-PA and cell migration: urokinase receptor as a ligand for a chemotactic G-protein-coupled receptor

FRANCESCO BLASI
Molecular Genetics Unit, Dept. of Cell Biology and Functional Genetics, Università Vita-Salute San Raffaele, Milan, Italy

Chemotaxis induced by u-PA requires the u-PA receptor (uPAR, CD87): it is exerted via an activated, soluble and cleaved, form of uPAR and is inhibited by pertussis toxin. The "activated" form of uPAR can be generated in vivo with uPA and in vitro with chymotrypsin (D2D388-274). We now report that the seven trans-membrane G-protein coupled receptor FPRL1/ALXR, a ubiquitously expressed receptor for Lipoxin A4, can mediate the chemotaxis induced by activated forms of uPAR.
HEK293 cells have no uPAR or FPRL1/ALXR. Transfection with FPRL1/ ALXR induces a chemotactic response to D2D388-274. In addition, an antibody against FPRL1/ ALXR inhibits specifically the chemotaxis induced by D2D388-274 in human peripheral blood monocytes, monocytes-derived immature dendritic cells and THP-1 cells. Pretreatment of the D2D388-274-sensitive THP-1 cells with a ligand of FPRL1/ ALXR (fMLP), results in desensitization. Conversely, pre-treatment of THP-1 cells with D2D388-274, desensitizes the cells to fMLP. FMLP pre-treatment also results in inhibition of the activation of the p54-p56 Hck induced by D2D388-274or by ATF in THP-1 cells. Finally, D2D388-274 specifically binds to THP-1 and FPRL1/ALXR expressing cells.

KARGER
Fax +41 61 306 12 34
E-Mail karger@karger.ch
www.karger.com

0301-0147/00/0309/0001$17.50/0

Accessible online at:
www.karger.com/journals/hae

Francesco Blasi
Unità di Genetica Molecolare - DIBIT - Dipartimento di Biologia e Biotecnologia
Università Vita-Salute San Raffaele
Via Olgettina, 58 - 20132 MILANO - ITALY
Tel. +39/02/26434832-44 - Fax +39/02/26434844
blasi.francesco@hsr.it

Hæmostasis

Lectures

Haemostasis 2001;31(suppl. 1):60-63

Properties and function of heparanase in cancer metastasis and angiogenesis

ISREAL VLODAVSKY, ORIT GOLDSHMIDT*
Department of Oncology, Hadassah-Hebrew University Hospital, Jerusalem, Israel

Abstract

Cleavage of heparan sulfate proteoglycans affects the integrity and functional state of tissues and thereby fundamental normal and pathological phenomena involving cell migration and response to changes in the extracellular microenvironment.

Heparanase, degrading heparan sulfate (HS) at specific intrachain sites, is synthesized as a latent ~65 kDa protein that is processed at the N-terminus into a highly active ~50 kDa form. The heparanase enzyme is preferentially expressed in human tumors and its overexpression in low-metastatic tumor cells confers a highly invasive phenotype in experimental animals. Heparanase also releases angiogenic factors and accessory fragments of HS from the tumor microenvironment and induces an angiogenic response in vivo. These effects were best demonstrated when the enzyme was secreted and/or expressed on the cell surface. Heparanase may thus facilitate tumor cell invasion, vascularization and survival, all critical events in cancer progression. These observations, the anti-cancerous effect of heparanase-inhibiting molecules, and the unexpected identification of a single predominant functional heparanase suggest that the enzyme is a promising target for drug development.

Introduction

Heparan sulfate proteoglycans (HSPGs) are ubiquitous macromolecules associated with the cell surface and ECM of a wide range of cells of vertebrate and invertebrate tissues [1, 2]. The basic HSPG structure consists of a protein core to which several linear heparan sulfate (HS) chains are covalently O-linked. The polysaccharide chains are typically composed of repeating hexuronic and D-glucosamine disaccharide units that are modified at various positions by sulfation, epimerization and N-acetylation, yielding clusters of sulfated disaccharides separated by low or non-sulfated regions [1, 2]. HS binds to and assembles ECM proteins and is playing important roles in cell-cell and cell-ECM interactions. Moreover, the HS chains, unique in their ability to bind a multitude of proteins, ensure that a wide variety of bioactive molecules bind to the cell surface and ECM and thereby function in the control of normal and pathological processes, among which are morphogenesis, tissue repair, inflammation, vascularization, and cancer metastasis [1-3]. Apart of sequestration of bioactive molecules, transmembrane (syndecans) and phospholipid-anchored (glypicans) HSPGs have a co-receptor role in which the proteoglycan, in concert with the other cell surface molecules, comprises a functional receptor complex that binds the ligand and mediates its action [1-3].

Molecular and biochemical properties.

Despite of earlier reports on the existence of several distinct mammalian HS degrading endoglycosidases (heparanases), the cloning of a single gene by several groups suggests that mammalian cells express primarily a single dominant functional heparanase enzyme [4-6]. The HS chains are cleaved by heparanase at only a few sites, resulting in HS fragments of still appreciable size (10–20 sugar units). The heparanase cDNA contains an open reading frame of 1629 bp that encodes for a 61.2 kDa polypeptide of 543 aminoacids. The mature active 50 kDa enzyme, isolated from cells and tissues, has its N-terminus 157 amino acids downstream from the initiation codon [4-6], suggesting post-translational processing of the heparanase polypeptide. Processing and activation occur during incubation of the full-length 65 kDa recombinant enzyme with several normal and transformed cells [6]. The nature of the cellular, apparently membrane bound enzyme(s), involved in activation of the latent heparanase has not been characterized. Site-directed mutagenesis revealed that similar to other glycosyl hydrolases, heparanase has a common catalytic mechanism that

KARGER

Fax +41 61 306 12 34
E-Mail karger@karger.ch
www.karger.com

0301-0147/00/0309/0001$17.50/0

Accessible online at:
www.karger.com/journals/hae

Isreal Vlodavsky
Deaprtment of Oncology - Hadassah - Hebrew University Hospital
POB 12000 - Jerusalem 91120 - ISRAEL
Tel. +972/2/6776776 - Fax +972/2/6422794
vlodavsk@cc.huji.ac.il

involves two conserved acidic residues, a putative proton donor at Glu225 and a nucleophile at Glu343 [7].

Involvement of heparanase in cancer progression

Preferential expression in human tumors.

Expression of the human heparanase mRNA in normal tissues is restricted primarily to the placenta and lymphoid organs [4-6]. Expression of the heparanase gene and protein was detected at early stages of human colon carcinoma progression, already at the stage of adenoma, while the adjacent normal-looking colonic tissue showed no expression of the enzyme [5]. Human mammary carcinoma expressed the heparanase mRNA and protein in both the in situ and invasive components of ductal and lobular origins. Normal breast tissue expressed little or no heparanase [5, 6]. Preferential expression of the heparanase mRNA and protein was also clearly demonstrated in tissue specimens derived from adenocarcinoma of the ovary, metastatic melanoma, oral squamous cell carcinoma, hepatocellular carcinoma and carcinomas of prostate, bladder, intestine and pancreas [5-7]. Patients exhibiting high levels of the heparanase mRNA in intestinal, bladder and pancreatic cancer tissues had a significantly shorter postoperative survival time than patients whose tumors contained relatively low levels of heparanase [7].

Angiogenesis.

HSPGs and HSPG-degrading enzymes have long been implicated in a number of angiogenesis-related cellular events, including cell invasion, migration, adhesion, differentiation and proliferation [1-3]. It appears that apart of direct involvement in BM invasion by EC, heparanase elicits an indirect angiogenic response by releasing HS-bound angiogenic growth factors (i.e., bFGF, VEGF) from ECM and BM, and by generating HS fragments which can potentiate bFGF receptor binding, dimerization and signaling. Using the mouse matrigel plug angiogenesis assay, we observed an increased angiogenic response to heparanase transfected T lymphoma cells, embedded in Matrigel and implanted subcutaneously, vs. a small or no response to the parental mock transfected cells [8]. Increased tissue vascularity was also observed in a mouse wound-healing model in response to a topical administration of recombinant heparanase [8].

Metastasis.

The ability of HSPGs to interact with various ECM macromolecules and with different attachment sites on plasma membranes suggests a key role for this proteoglycan in the self-assembly and insolubility of ECM components, as well as in cell adhesion and locomotion [1, 2]. Cleavage of HS may therefore result in disassembly of the subendothelial ECM and play a significant role in extravasation of blood-borne cells. Expression of heparanase correlates with the metastatic potential of human tumor cells [4-6]. Moreover, elevated levels of heparanase were detected in the urine of some patients with aggressive metastatic disease. Evidence for a direct role of heparanase in tumor metastasis was provided by the increased lung and liver metastasis of mouse B16 melanoma and T-lymphoma cells following transfection and overexpression of the heparanase gene [6].

Cell surface expression and secretion of heparanase.

We have recently cloned a chicken heparanase that unlike the human enzyme is readily secreted and preferentially associated with the cell surface [9]. Cells transfected with the chicken enzyme, or with a chimeric construct composed of the human enzyme fused to the chicken heparanase signal sequence, exhibited a higher angiogenic and metastatic potential, as compared with cells overexpressing the human enzyme, indicating that cellular localization of heparanase plays a decisive role in tumor progression. Mice inoculated with lymphoma cells expressing the secreted enzyme succumb because of liver metastasis and dysfunction, already when the primary tumor was small and did not exceed 1% of the body weight. Similarly, we have demonstrated a remarkable pro-angiogenic response to cells over-expressing the secreted enzyme relative to cells expressing the heparanase enzyme primarily intracellularly (Goldshmidt et al., submitted).

Inhibitory molecules.

Non-anticoagulant species of heparin and various sulfated polysaccharides which inhibited experimental metastasis, also inhibited tumor cell heparanase, while other related compounds had a small or no effect on both parameters [4, 5]. Regardless of the mode of action, heparin also appears to have a beneficial effect in cancer patients. Inhibition of both heparanase activity and experimental metastasis was exerted by heparin species containing >14 sugar units and having sulfate groups at both the N and O positions. While O-desulfation abolished the inhibitory effect of heparin, O-sulfated, N-substituted (e.g., N-acetyl or N-hexanoyl) species of low molecular weight heparin

retained a high inhibitory activity [10]. Potent inhibition of heparanase activity and tumor metastasis was also obtained with other sulfated polysaccharides (i.e., laminaran sulfate) and heparin-mimicking polyanionic molecules, although an effect on selectin mediated cell adhesion could not be excluded.
The oligosaccharide chain length and degree of sulfation were more important parameters than the sugar composition and type of linkage.
Phosphomannopentaose sulfate (PI-88) and maltohexaose sulfate were comparable to heparin in their heparanase inhibiting activity [4]. PI-88 is being evaluated in a multi-center clinical trial [4]. Although heparanase-inhibiting compounds might interfere with normal functions of the enzyme (e.g., immune surveillance, tissue repair and remodeling, HS turnover), heparanase is an attractive drug target. It is hoped that identification of the sugar residues in HS adjacent to the heparanase cleavage site, as well as crystalization and analysis of the 3D-structure of the enzyme will lead to a rational design of highly specific heparanase inhibitors. Heparanase is the first mammalian HS-degrading enzyme that has been cloned, expressed and characterized. This may lead to identification and cloning of other members of a putative family of mammalian glycosaminoglycan degrading enzymes (e.g., chondroitinase, dermatanase, keratanase), toward a better understanding of the function and biological significance of both the enzymes and their polysaccharide substrates.

Figure 1. *Scheme of the human heparanase gene and protein.*

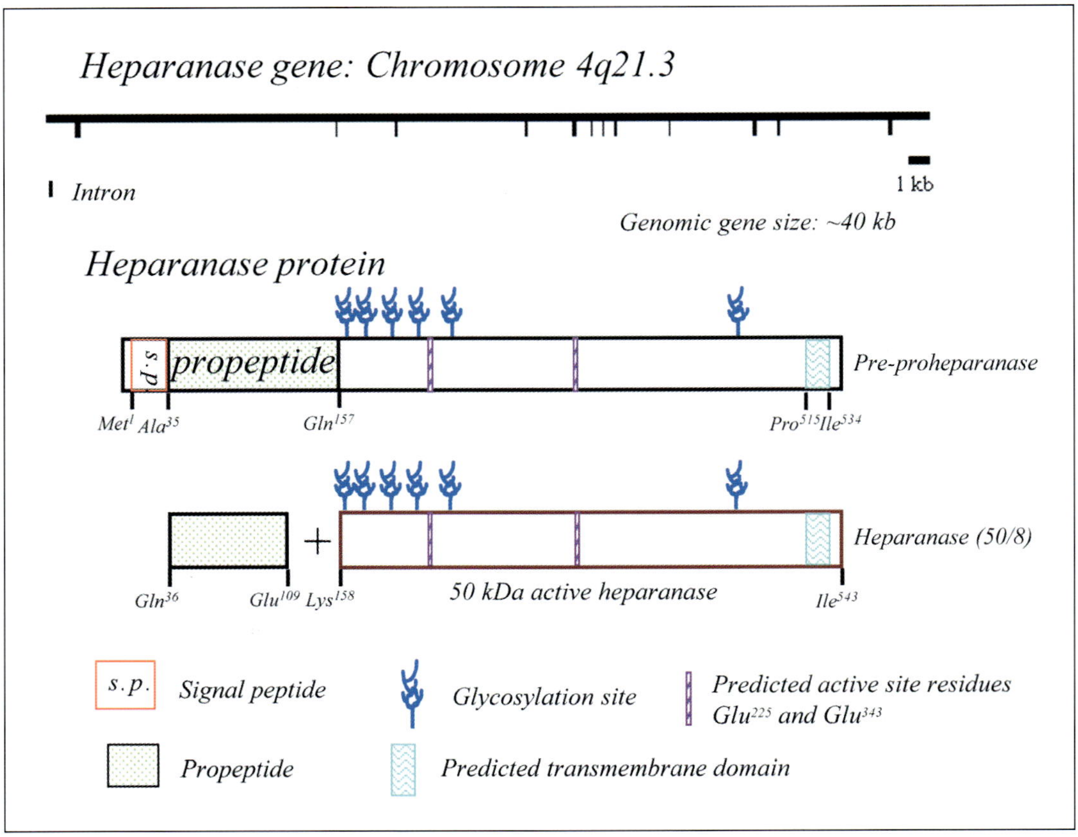

References

1. Esko JD, Lindahl U. Molecular diversity of heparan sulfate. J Clin Invest 2001; 108 :169-173.
2. Iozzo RV, San Antonio JD. Heparan sulfate proteoglycans: Heavy hitters in the angiogenesis arena from molecular design to cellular function. J Clin Invest 2001; 108: 349-355.
3. Vlodavsky I, Miao H-Q, Medalion B, Danagher P, Ron D. Involvement of heparan sulfate and related molecules in sequestration and growth promoting activity of fibroblast growth factor. Cancer Metastasis Rev 1996; 15: 177-186.
4. Parish CR, Freeman C, Hulett MD. Heparanase: a key enzyme involved in cell invasion. Biochim Biophys Acta 2001; 1471: M99-M108.
5. Vlodavsky I, Friedmann Y. Molecular properties and function of heparanase in cancer metastasis and angiogenesis. J Clin Invest 2001; 108: 341-347.
6. Vlodavsky I, Friedmann Y, Elkin M, Aingorn H, Atzmon R, Ishai-Michaeli R, Bitan M, Pappo O, Peretz T, Michal I, Spector L, Pecker I. Mammalian heparanase: gene cloning, expression and function in tumor progression and metastasis. Nat Med 1999; 5: 793-802.
7. Gohji K, Hirano H, Okamoto M, Kitazawa S, Toyoshima M, Dong J, Katsuoka Y, Nakajima M. Expression of three extracellular matrix degradative enzymes in bladder cancer. Int J Cancer 2001; 95: 295-301.
8. Elkin M, Ishai-Michaeli R, Friedmann Y, Papo O, Pecker I, Vlodavsky I. Heparanase as mediator of angiogenesis: mode of action. FASEB J 2001; 10.1096/fj.00-0895fje
9. Goldshmidt O, Zcharia E, Aingorn H, Guatta-Rangini Z, Atzmon R, Michal I Pecker I, Mitrani E, Vlodavsky I. Secretion and expression pattern of human and chicken heparanases are determined by their signal peptide sequences. J Biol Chem 2001; 276: 29178-29187.
10. Vlodavsky I, Moshen M, Lider O, Svahn CM, Ekre HP, Vigoda M, Ishai-Michaeli R, Peretz T. Inhibition of tumor metastasis by heparanase inhibiting species of heparin. Invasion & Metastasis 1994; 14: 290-302.

Hæmostasis

Lectures

Haemostasis 2001;31(suppl. 1):64-66

Platelets cross-talk with tumor cells

DAVID VARON*, ALEXANDER BRILL
Coagulation Unit, Department of Hematology, Hadassah, Hebrew University Medical Center, Jerusalem, Israel.

The potential role, of platelets in tumor metastasis was first suggested by Gasic and co-workers thirty three years ago, when they demonstrated an anti-metastatic effect of platelet reduction in an experimental animal model [1]. This pioneering work stimulated several laboratories, including ours, to study different aspects of platelet tumor-cell interactions.

In this review we will discuss three aspects of the subject including a) Direct interaction between platelet and tumor cells (TC), b) Mechanisms of tumor cell adhesion and migration through the vessel wall and, c) The role of platelets in angiogenesis.

Direct platelet interaction with tumor cells

Early works by Karpatkin and his group have demonstrated the ability of several tumor cell lines to induce in vitro platelet aggregation [2]. In their studies they identified mechanisms, which are involved in this interaction including complement and thrombin mediated processes among others. They concluded that different TCs interact with platelets via different mechanisms. Similar results were reported by others, confirming the role of calcium and calcium channels as well as of tissue factor, derived from TCs, in the activation of platelets and the coagulation cascade [3,4]. In our laboratory we studied the potential role of platelet activating factor (PAF), in this interaction. We observed the inhibitory effect of a PAF antagonist on platelet aggregation induced by several TC lines (unpublished data). However, when anti-aggregating agents were tested for their potential anti metastatic effect, only in vitro but not in vivo inhibition was observed [5]. Therefore alternative mechanisms, by which platelets might mediate tumor metastasis were sought.

The potential role of platelets as an adhesion substrate for TCs during the metastatic process was investigated in vitro. These works have established that many TC lines adhere to platelets via the integrin receptor GPIIb-IIIa interaction with it's ligands, fibronectin and von Willebrand Factor (vWF) [6]. This adhesion is enhanced by pre-treatment of both platelets and TCs with thrombin, suggesting that activation of platelets and TCs plays a role in this interaction. All of these observations were confirmed in vivo, demonstrating the role of platelet GPIIb-IIIa, vWF, fibronectin and thrombin in tumor metastasis [6]. An alternate mechanism by which TC interact with platelets was described by Varki and co-workers. They demonstrated that sialylated fucosylated antigens on TC surface, mediate adhesion to platelets via interaction with p-selectin. This conclusion was supported, by both in vitro and by in vivo studies using P-selecting "knockout" mice [7].

Tumor cell adhesion and migration through the vessel wall

In order to cross the vessel wall in the process of hematogenous spread, TCs must interact with both endothelial cells (EC), and the subendothelial extracellular matrix (ECM). In our laboratory, we studied adhesion properties of human TC lines to both EC and ECM, under flow conditions, and evaluated the potential role for platelets in these interactions. Our studies established that thrombin activated platelets mediate TC adhesion to EC. We confirmed that the adhesion of activated platelets to the EC is mediated by P-selectin and GPIIb-IIIa while the interaction between TC to the adherent platelets is mediated by GPIIb-IIIa alone [8]. We also demonstrated that TC adhesion to ECM under flow is platelet dependent, and that this interaction is mediated by platelet GPIIb-IIIa and by the TC av integrin regardless of the b subunit [9]. These studies have suggested that TCs may induce thrombin generation via surface tissue factor or cancer procoagulant, and that thrombin might mediate TC interaction with both platelets and EC.

KARGER
Fax +41 61 306 12 34
E-Mail karger@karger.ch
www.karger.com

0301-0147/00/0309/0001$17.50/0

Accessible online at:
www.karger.com/journals/hae

David Varon
Coagulation Unit - Department of Hematology
Hadassah-Hebrew University Medical Center - P.O. Box 12000
Jerusalem 91120 - ISRAEL
Tel. +972/2/6777672 - Fax +972/2/6449580
dvaron@bezeqint.net

Direct adhesion of TC to EC was also demonstrated in another study, which suggested that this interaction is thrombin mediated [6].

An additional role, for platelets in TC invasion, was suggested by Vlodavsky and his group. They have shown that platelets can facilitate tumor invasion via heparanase degradation of the ECM [10]. This group has established that platelets are a major source of heparanase, and that heparanase can be activated by a yet to be discovered cleaving protease. Tumor cells were found to induce heparanase activation, and to express heparanase activity, which is correlated with the invasiveness of the specific type of tumor [11,12].

The role of platelets in angiogenesis

The involvement of angiogenesis in tumor growth is well established since early works by Folkman and others [13]. Platelets were recently found to release, upon activation, VEGF and PDGF, which play an important role in the angiogenic process [13]. Other investigators have reported that VEGF alone can induce vWF expression/release from resting EC, thus promoting platelet adhesion and colonization of TC by itself. In addition, activated platelets release platelet factor-4 and express thrombospondin, both of which were found to inhibit angiogenesis. Recently, activated platelet-released phospholipids, (including sphingosine 1-phosphate, SPP, and others), were found to induce both EC changes associated with angiogenesis, and to enhance chemoattractive activity of EC during thrombosis. These observations suggest that SPP and other platelet-derived lipid mediators may provide another link between hemostasis and angiogenesis [14].

Taken together, the above observations suggest that platelets may participate in angiogenesis in many different ways, including both promoting and inhibitory effects. The physiological importance of each of these effects as well as of the net contribution of platelets to angiogenesis is yet to be established.

Conclusions

Platelets cross-talk with TC via different mechanisms, including TC induction of platelet activation, TC adhesion to platelets and others. Platelets were found to facilitate TC adhesion and migration through the vessel wall by a variety of mechanisms including bridging between TC and EC under both static and flow conditions and by allowing migration of TC through the ECM by heparanase activity.

Platelets may also be found to play a modulating role in angiogenesis, which is a crucial step in tumor growth. Thus future perspectives for research as well as for drug discovery in this field appear quite exciting.

References

1. Gasic GJ, Gasic TB, Stewart CC. Antimetastatic effects associated with platelet reduction. Proc Natl Acad Sci 1968; 61:46-52.
2. Lerner WA, Pearlstein E, Ambrogio C. Karpatkin S. A new mechanism for tumor-induced platelet aggregation. Int J Cancer 1983; 31: 463-469.
3. Timar J, Chopra H, Rong X. et al. Calcium channel blocker treatment of tumor cells induces alterations in the cytoskeleton. J Cancer Res Clin Oncol. 1992; 118 (6): 425-434.
4. Bastida E, Ordinas A, Escolar G, Jamieson GA. Tissue factor in microvesicles shed from U87MG human glioblastoma cells induces coagulation, platelet aggregation, and thrombogenesis. Blood 1984; 64 (1): 177-184.
5. Karpatkin S, Pearlstein E, Ambrogio C, Coller BS. Role of adhesive proteins in platelet tumor interaction in vitro and metastasis formation in vivo. J Clin Invest 1988; 81 (4): 1012-1019.
6. Nierodzik ML, Klepfish A, Karpatkin S. Role of platelets, thrombin, integrin IIb-IIIa, fibronectin and von Willebrand Factor in tumor adhesion in vitro and metastasis in vivo. Thromb Haemost 1995; 74 (1): 282-290.
7. Varki A, Varki NM. P-selectin, carcinoma metastasis and heparin: novel mechanistic connections with therapeutic implications. Braz J Med Biol Res. 2001; 34 (6): 711-717.
8. Dardik R, Savion N, Kaufmann Y, Varon D. Thrombin promotes platelet-mediated melanoma cell adhesion to endothelia cells under flow conditions: role of platelet GP P-selectin and GPIIb-IIIa. Brit J Cancer Res. 1998; 77 (12): 2069-2077.
9. Dardik R, Kaufmann Y, Savion N, Rosenberg N, Shenkman B, Varon D. Platelet mediate tumor cell adhesion to the subendothelium under flow conditions: Involvement of platelet GPIIb-IIIa and tumor cell _v integrins. Int J Cancer. 1997; 70: 201-207.
10. Eldor A, Bar-Ner M, Yahalom J, Fuks Z, Vlodavsky I. Role of heparanase in platelet and tumor cell interaction with the subendothelial extracellular matrix. Semin Thromb Hemost. 1987; 13 (4): 475-488.
11. Haimovitz-Friedman A, Falcon DJ, Eldoe A, Schirrmacher V, Vlodavsky I, Fux Z. Activation of platelet heparitinase by tumor cell-derived factors. Blood. 1991; 78 (3): 789-796.
12. Vlodavsky I, Friedmann Y. Molecular properties and involvement of heparanase in cancer metastasis and angiogenesis. JCI. 2001; 108 (3); 341-347.
13. Pinedo HM, Verheul HMW, D'Amato RJ, Folkman J. Involvement of platelets in tumor angiogenesis? Lancet. 1998; 352: 1775-1777.
14. English D, Garcia JG, Brindley DN. Platelet-released phospho lipids link haemostasis and angiogenesis. Cardiovasc Res. 2001; 49 (3): 588-599.

Hæmostasis

Lectures

Haemostasis 2001;31(suppl. 1):67

Prevention and treatment of VTE in cancer

An overview of thromboprophylaxis in malignancy

AJAY K. KAKKAR
Imperial College, London, UK

Venous thromboembolism (VTE) is increasingly recognised to be an important complication of cancer therapy whether it be associated with surgical intervention, chemo or radiotherapy and with the use of central venous catheters.

The immobilised cancer patient confined to bed is nearly twice as likely to die of pulmonary embolism than his non-cancer counterpart.

The risk of thromboembolic disease varies with cancer type. Methods advocated for the prevention of VTE in the cancer patients include mechanical methods such as compression stockings and pneumatic calf compression, and pharmacological methods which include low dose unfractionated heparin (uFH), low molecular weight heparin (LMWH) and oral anticoagulants.

The evaluation of efficacy and safety of these different methods has not been assessed to the same extent in medical and surgical cancer patients. The most compelling evidence is from studies of either low dose or low molecular weight heparin in cancer surgical patients. The duration of primary prophylaxis against cancer associated VTE has yet to be defined, although in those undergoing major abdominal or pelvic operations for malignancy recent evidence suggests that prolonged prophylaxis with LMWH post discharge from hospital will significantly reduce late complications from deep vein thrombosis.

Prevention of VTE in cancer patients represents an important challenge since cancer patients experiencing a thrombotic episode have a poor outcome with greater probability of death. In addition to the prevention of thrombotic disease antithrombotic therapy with LMWH may prolong survival in cancer patients although the mechanisms for this action remain unclear, and have yet to establish in prospective clinical trials.

KARGER

Fax +41 61 306 12 34
E-Mail karger@karger.ch
www.karger.com

0301-0147/00/0309/0001$17.50/0

Accessible online at:
www.karger.com/journals/hae

Ajay K. Kakkar
Hammersmith Hospital - Imperial College
Thrombosis Research Institute - Emmanuel Kaye Bldg
Manresa Rd Chelsea - London England SW3 6LR - UK
Tel. +44/20/73518309 - Fax +44/20/73518317
akkakkar@tri-london.ac.uk

Hæmostasis

Lectures

Haemostasis 2001;31(suppl. 1):68-69

Management of thromboembolic disease in cancer patients

MARK N. LEVINE
McMaster University, Hamilton, Ontario, Canada

Patients with malignant disease have a high risk of thromboembolism. The pathogenesis of thromboembolism in cancer patients is multifactorial [1]. These include procoagulants produced by tumour cells, immobilization, surgery, anticancer drugs and indwelling venous catheters. The occurrence of thrombosis in the cancer patient complicates their management [2].

In general, the objectives of treating patients with venous thromboembolism are to prevent death from pulmonary embolism, to reduce morbidity from the acute event, to minimize post-phlebitic symptoms and to prevent thromboembolic pulmonary hypertension. However, the physician sometimes may have to decide whether to treat venous thromboembolism in a patient with terminal malignant disease.
In such circumstances, treatment may help palliate the symptoms of acute venous thromboembolism. For example, painful swelling of the leg and dyspnea and chest pain from pulmonary embolism.

Cancer patients with established venous thrombosis are more likely to develop recurrent venous thromboembolism than non-cancer patients with thrombosis [3]. Low molecular weight heparins have replaced standard unfractionated heparin as the initial treatment for acute venous thromboembolism. Low molecular weight heparin does not require laboratory monitoring. In a number of randomized trials, low molecular weight heparin administered subcutaneously on a weight-adjusted basis has been shown to be as safe and effective as standard unfractionated heparin administered by continuous intravenous infusion for the treatment of acute proximal deep vein thrombosis (DVT) in hospitalized patients [4]. Clinical trials in patients with acute proximal DVT (including cancer patients) have demonstrated that patients can be treated safely at home with subcutaneous low molecular weight heparin without admission to hospital [5-7].

Patients with DVT who are treated with an initial course of heparin therapy require continuing anticoagulant therapy to prevent recurrence. Vitamin K antagonists have been shown to be effective in preventing recurrent thrombosis in patients with established thromboembolism. Warfarin is the standard long term anticoagulant therapy for patients with venous thromboembolism. Warfarin therapy should be monitored to maintain the INR between 2.0 and 3.0. However, such therapy may not be optimal in cancer patients for a number of reasons. Poor nutrition, infection, concomitant medications and impaired hepatic function can cause unpredictable changes in the dose response of oral anticoagulants. In addition, temporary cessation of anticoagulant therapy may be needed to accommodate chemotherapy-induced thrombocytopenia and invasive procedures. Cancer patients are also considered to be at increased risk of recurrent thromboembolism and anticoagulant related bleeding compared to non-cancer patients [3]. Clinical trials are evaluating low molecular weight heparins for long term therapy in cancer patients with venous thromboembolism. In cancer patients, the duration of anticoagulant therapy should be at least six months or longer; i.e. as long as the malignant disease is active.

Cancer patients who develop a documented recurrent thrombosis while on therapeutic oral anticoagulant therapy represent a difficult therapeutic challenge. There are several options after retreatment of the acute episode with heparin (or low molecular weight heparin). These include continued oral anticoagulant therapy with warfarin (but at a higher targeted INR), adjusted dose

KARGER
Fax +41 61 306 12 34
E-Mail karger@karger.ch
www.karger.com

0301-0147/00/0309/0001$17.50/0

Accessible online at:
www.karger.com/journals/hae

Mark N. Levine
McMaster University - Faculty of Health Sciences, RM 2E22
1200 Main Street West - Hamilton Ontario - CANADA L8N 3Z5
Tel. +1/905/3894411 42176 - Fax +1/905/3899288
mlevine@fhs.csu.mcmaster.ca

subcutaneous heparin to maintain a therapeutic APTT or weight-adjusted low molecular weigh heparin. In patients at high risk for pulmonary embolism, an inferior vena caval filter can be inserted in addition to the above measures. The use of an inferior vena caval filter alone should only be used in patients with active bleeding or at very high risk of bleeding. In a randomized trial, the use of a vena caval filter reduced the rate of recurrent pulmonary embolism over the short-term, but at the expense of recurrent deep vein [8].

References

1. Rickles FR, Levine MN. Venous thromboembolism in malignancy and malignancy in venous thromboembolism. Haemostasis 1998; 28 (suppl 3):43-49.
2. Lee AYY, Levine MN. Management of venous thromboembolism in cancer patients. Oncology 2000; 14:409-421.
3. Hutten BA, Prins MH, Gent M, Ginsberg J, Tijssen J, Buller HR. Incidence of recurrent thromboembolic and bleeding complications among patients with venous thromboembolism in relation to both malignancy and achieved International Normalized Ratio: a retrospective analysis. J Clin Oncol 2000;18:3078-83.
4. Weitz J. Low molecular weight heparins. New England Journal of Medicine 1997; 337:688-691.
5. Levine M, Gent M, Hirsh J, et al. A comparison of low molecular weight heparin administered primarily at home with unfractionated heparin administered in the hospital for proximal deep vein thrombosis. N Engl J Med 1996; 334:677-681.
6. Koopman MW, Prandoni P, Piovella F, et al. Treatment of venous thrombosis with intravenous unfractionated heparin administered in the hospital as compared with subcutaneous low molecular weight heparin administered at home. N Engl J Med 1996; 334:682-687.
7. The Columbus Investigators. Low molecular weight heparin in the treatment of patients with venous thromboembolism. N Engl J Med. 1997;337:657-662.
8. Decousus H, Leizorovicz A, Parent F, et al. A clinical trial of vena caval filters in the prevention of pulmonary embolism in patients with proximal deep-vein thrombosis. Prevention du Risque d'Emblie Pulmonaire par Interruption Cave Study Group. N Engl J Med 1998; 38:409-415.

Hæmostasis

Vol. 31, Suppl. 1, 2001

Abstracts

Hæmostasis

Oral Communications

Haemostasis 2001;31(suppl. 1):72-77

OC 01
Promotion of Factor Xa and Thrombin Generation by T Lymphoblastoid Cell Lines

TW BARROWCLIFFE [1], P FABREGAS [2], J CANCELAS [2], M RABANEDA [2], W PICKERING [1], E GRAY [1], J FELEZ [2]
[1]NIBSC Potters Bar, UK, & [2]Institut de Recerca Oncologica, Barcelona, Spain.

Procoagulant activity (PCA) of leukocytes due to expression of tissue factor (TF) is well known, but PCA due to expression of negatively charged phospholipids (PL) is less described. We have characterised the PCA of six well-established cell lines by assays of TF, thrombin generation and FXa generation, by flow cytometry using Annexin V, and by binding studies with Factors VIII and IXa. The monocytic (THP-1 & U937) and promyelocytic (NB4) cells expressed high concentrations of TF antigen and activity, whereas TF in the lymphocytic cells (Molt 4, Jurkat & Nalm 6) was very low or absent. However, the T-lymphoblastoid cells (Molt 4 & Jurkat) promoted the generation of large amounts of thrombin despite their low TF content, and these cells were also the most active in supporting Factor Xa generation. Molt 4 cells bound Factors VIII and IXa with high capacity and Annexin V inhibited activity of these and other cell lines in both FXa generation and TF assays. These results indicate that the PCA of T-lymphoblastoid lines is due to expression of negatively charged phospholipids. Flow cytometry studies showed Annexin V binding to the major population of non-apoptotic Molt 4 cells and the PCA of Molt 4 was not increased when apoptosis was induced by staurosporine, indicating that PCA is independent of apoptotic status. These studies emphasise the important role of negatively charged phospholipids in promoting the generation of Factor Xa and thrombin in T lymphoblastoid cell lines.

OC 02
Shear Stress Activation of Huvec Modulates the Adhesion of Tumour Cells to the Vessel Wall

*F FAUVEL-LAFEVE, N GOMES, J VASSY, C LEGRAND**
U553 INSERM and LAIPC, Hôpital Saint Louis, Paris, France

The interactions between tumour cells, endothelial cells and the extracellular matrix (ECM) are involved in tumour cell extravasation and subsequent metastasis. We have studied the adhesion of breast adenocarcinoma cells (MDA-MB-231) to human umbilical vein endothelial cells (HUVEC) and their ECM in whole blood and under flow conditions. This study was done on HUVEC grown on coverslips under static conditions and then conditioned in flow for two hours at shear stress (t) of 5 (t5) and 13 (t13) dynes/cm^2. HUVEC submitted to flow were activated. In each case, HUVEC matrix was obtained after the lysis of cells by 0.1% NH_4OH. Coverslips coated by HUVEC, either kept under static conditions or submitted to flow as above, or the corresponding matrices were placed in a parallel plate perfusion chamber and perfused with heparin anticoagulated blood containing In111 labelled MDA-MB-231 cells. MDA-MB-231 adhesion to endothelial cells or their ECM was studied at two shear rates, 300 and 1500 sec^{-1} corresponding to the shear conditions respectively observed in medium and small sized arteries. MDA-MB-231 adhesion to endothelial cells was independent of perfusate shear rate, whereas a shear rate of 1500 sec^{-1} enhanced tumour cell adhesion to the ECM. Moreover, MDA-MB-231 adhered preferentially to t5 pre-conditioned HUVEC perfused at 1500 sec^{-1} or t13 HUVEC perfused at 300 sec-1. This indicates that in the circulation, tumour cells preferentially adhere to endothelial cells submitted to flow perturbations. A double labelling using pancytoketatin and anti-$\alpha2\beta3$ antibodies to respectively label tumour cells and platelets showed that, on HUVEC, adherent tumour cells were isolated and small platelets aggregates were present at the proximity of tumour cells. On the matrix, aggregates formed by platelets and tumour cells were observed suggesting that platelets first adhere to the matrix and then aggregate with tumour cells. However, on the endothelium, MDA-MB-231 adhered directly to HUVEC and this interaction could activate HUVEC and tumour cells and induce platelet aggregation. Thus, the arrest of tumour cells in the microvasculature is not only due to an occlusion of small vessels by tumour cells, but to a specific interaction of tumour cells with the endothelium.

OC 03
Inhibition of TF Activity Reduces Network Formation in an In Vitro Model of Angiogenesis

NJ JAMES [1], C ETTELAIE [2], AND KR BRUCKDORFER [1]*

[1]Dept. of Biochemistry and Molecular Biology, RF&UCMS, London, and [2]Biomedical Section, Dept. of Biological Science, University of Hull, Cottingham Road, Hull, UK

T24 bladder carcinoma cells grown on Engelbreth Holm Swarm mouse sarcoma basement membrane matrix form a network of tubules. TF activity in the culture system was inhibited by either using an antibody, or using a peptide. The TF85G9 antibody exhibits an inhibitory activity towards TF [1]. The peptide (KRAD14) is derived from the LDL receptor-binding region of apo B100. We have previously demonstrated that the KRAD14 peptide is a potent inhibitor of the procoagulant activity of TF [2]. Treatment of cultures with the TF85G9 antibody and the KRAD14 peptide lead to a concentration-dependent reduction in the density of cellular networks. These results demonstrate that the activity of TF has a role in determining the density of network formation in these cultures. Furthermore, these results show that the KRAD14 peptide inhibits network formation more efficiently that the TF85G9 antibody (IC50, 1 & 30 μM respectively). A stable structure based upon the KRAD14 peptide could prove effective in the treatment of disease states where the pathology is promoted by neoangiogenesis e.g. tumour metastasis and atherosclerosis. Since the KRAD14 peptide is much smaller than the TF85G9 antibody Fab fragments, it may be more suitable for use in targeted drug delivery applications e.g. microsomal delivery.

1-Ruf, W. et al Biochem J. 278, 729 (1991)
2- Ettelaie, C. et al. Biochem. J. 333, 433 (1998)

OC 04
The Risk of Venous Thrombosis in Cancer Patients With or Without the Factor V Leiden Mutation

JW BLOM, CJM DOGGEN, FR ROSENDAAL*

Leiden University Medical Center, Department of Clinical Epidemiology, Leiden, The Netherlands

Cancer is an important risk factor for venous thrombosis. A recent case control study has shown a relative risk of 4.1 in cancer patients compared to the general population (Heit, Arch Intern Med. 2000;160: 809-15). Also the factor V Leiden mutation is a (genetic) risk factor for venous thrombosis (Bertina, Thromb Haemost 1995,74:449-53). Due to thrombosis being a multicausal disease, it is expected that the interaction between cancer and the factor V Leiden mutation will lead to clinical venous thrombosis. To study the interaction of cancer with the factor V Leiden mutation on the occurrence of thrombosis, we conducted a case-control study among patients with a first event of deep venous thrombosis of the leg or arm, or of pulmonary embolism before the age of 80 years. Cases were identified in five different anticoagulation clinics, starting from March 1999. Their partners were asked to participate as controls. All participants filled in a questionnaire on risk factors for thrombosis. A part of the questionnaire included questions on cancer, date of diagnosis, type and treatment. Three months after the discontinuation of the oral anticoagulation both cases and controls were invited to give a blood sample. In the first year we included 1267 patients (verification of diagnosis pending) and 713 control subjects. One hundred and fortytwo (142) patients died because of cancer, and 40 were in a terminal stage before inclusion and thus could not participate. The factor V Leiden mutation has been measured in 1586 participants. The questionnaires (1865) have been processed. Factor V Leiden mutation increased the risk of venous thrombosis 2.9 times (CI 95%: 1.9 - 4.4), cancer increased the risk 2.7 times (CI 95%: 1.9 – 4.0). The table shows the risk in the presence of combinations of the factor V Leiden mutation and cancer. Although the risk of venous thrombosis was highest in cancer patients with factor V Leiden mutation, no interactive effect was observed, i.e., the joint effect was not higher than the sum of the separate effects.

Table to abstract OC04:

Factor V Leiden	Cancer	Cases	Controls	Odds ratio
-	-	717	484	1
-	+	92	27	2.3
+	-	119	26	3.1
+	+	15	2	5.1

OC 05
Malignant Disease Following Pre-Eclampsia: Preliminary Data from The Jerusalem Perinatal Study

*S HARLAP[1], E TIRAM[2], S MASSALHA[2], L DEUTSCH[2], A KNAANIE[2], Y FRIEDLANDER[2], O PALTIEL[2,3]**
[1]Dept. of Obstetrics and Gynecology and Kaplan Cancer Center, New York University School of Medicine, New York, NY, USA; [2]School of Public Health, Dept. of Social Medicine, Hadassah-Hebrew University, Jerusalem, Israel, [3]Dept of Hematology, Hadassah Medical Center, Jerusalem, Israel

Pre-eclampsia has been associated with genetic defects in coagulation, fibrinolysis and angiogenesis, among others. An Israeli study revealed that 56% of women with pre-eclampsia carried thrombophilic mutations (Kupferminc, Obstet Gynecol 2000;96:45-9). Previous studies have suggested a negative association with subsequent malignant disease, both in offspring and mothers. We studied malignancies reported to the Israel Cancer Registry, comparing 825 Jewish women diagnosed with pre-eclampsia versus 39,679 other mothers who gave birth in 1964-76 in the Jerusalem Perinatal Study. There were 2,547 first primary malignancies diagnosed before 1999, including 1,031 breast cancers. Using Cox proportional hazards methods to control for age, parity, immigration, measures of socio-economic status and ethnic origin, we found that women diagnosed with pre-eclampsia had an increased relative risk (RR) of subsequent breast cancer mortality (RR: 2.03; 95% confidence interval: 1.19-3.48), and breast cancer incidence (RR: 1.46; 95% CI: 1.02-2.09). Positive relations were found with stomach cancer (based on a small number of cases) and all cancers (RR: 1.31; 95% CI: 1.03-1.66). The association of breast cancer with pre-eclampsia was particularly evident in women of Near East origin (RR: 1.97; 95% CI: 1.13-3.44) as opposed to other ethnic groups. In the subset of 24,290 women followed from their first pregnancy, breast cancer mortality (RR: 2.57; 95% CI: 1.31-5.05) and incidence (RR: 1.99, 95% CI: 1.29-3.05) were also increased in the 467 with pre-eclampsia, as was all cancer incidence (RR 1.78; 95% CI: 1.32-2.41). Further investigations should be carried out to determine whether this association is mediated via thrombophilic mutations.

OC 06
Chemotherapy-Induced Activation of Hemostasis: Effects of a LMW Heparin (dalteparin sodium) on Plasma Markers of Hemostatic Activation

IC WEITZ, VK ISRAEL, JR WAISMAN, C PRESANT, L ROCHANDA, HA LIEBMAN*
USC Keck School of Medicine, Los Angeles, USA

Purpose: To evaluate the effect of standard chemotherapeutic regimens on the hemostatic profile of patients with breast and lung carcinoma, and to evaluate the effect of a single dose of a low molecular weight (LMW) heparin (dalteparin sodium) administered prior to the chemotherapy on markers of hemostatic activation. **Patients & Methods:** 11 patients with breast cancer and 10 patients with lung cancer receiving systemic chemotherapy were studied. Ten breast cancer patients and 9 lung cancer patients completed at least one cycle of treatment and had all hemostatic studies. Patients had a complete hemostatic andprothrombotic profile performed at study initiation. Markers of hemostatic activation consisting of immuno-assays for thrombin-antithrombin (TAT) complex and D-dimer were measured in plasma samples obtained prior to chemotherapy and at 1, 24 and 48 hours after treatment. An administration of 2500 U of dalteparin was given prior to the 2nd cycle of chemotherapy; 5000 U of dalteparin were given prior to the 4th treatment cycle. **Results:** Chemotherapy resulted in statistically significant increases in TAT and D-dimer for the 1, 24 and 48 hour plasma samples in both the breast and lung cancer patients for all cycles of chemotherapy given without LMW heparin. There were statistically significant increases in basal thrombin generation over the 4 cycles of treatment which was unrelated to active cancer. Both pretreatment doses of dalteparin effectively prevented increases in the markers of hemostatic activation. However, in the lung cancer patients, who had significantly increased basal thrombin generation, the 5000 U dalteparin dose was more effective. **Conclusion:** Chemotherapy results in significant hemostatic activation in patients with breast and lung cancer. The effect of treatment appears to be cumulative. A single dose of LMW heparin administered prior to therapy can suppress hemostatic activation.

OC 07
Two Years Experience with the Collagen-Binding Assay for Quantification of Von-Willebrand-Factor-Cleaving Protease (VWF-CP)

F BERGMANN[1], U SCHULER[2], G SIEGERT[1], D ANGERHAUS[1], R SCHNEPPENHEIM[3], U BUDDE[1]*
[1]Labassociation Prof. Arndt & Partner, Coagulation Laboratory, Hamburg, [2]University Hospital Dresden and [3]University Hospital Eppendorf, Hamburg, Germany

In patients with chronic thrombocytopenia the introduction of the VWF-CP assay is very helpful in classification of microangiopathic thrombocytopenia. However, recent reports doubt the specificity of the assay. The major advantage of the collagen binding assay is the fast turn-over time of only one day and it is less technical demanding than the originally described vWF-multimer analysis method by Furlan et al (NEJM 1998). Instead of a plasma preparation we use recombinant von Willebrand factor as the uncleaved substrate. Over a period of 2 years we analysed approximately 500 samples of patients with thrombocytopenia, including patients with TTP, HUS, HELLP-syndrome and patients after bone marrow transplantation (BMT). Additionally, we investigated 100 patients with metastatic solid tumors. In our opinion patients with TTP are characterized specifically by a complete absence of the VWF-CP due to an inhibitor in most of the non-familiar cases. Patients with HUS or women with HELLP-syndrome never showed a relevant decrease of the VWF-CP activity. Some patients after BMT had a considerably decreased activity but were always distinguishable from non-BMT-TTP-patients. In cancer patients we observed a decrease of the VWF-CP, but only in 2 of 100 patients the VWF-CP was completely absent. These data are in contrast to published data by Oleksowicz et al (CANCER RESEARCH 1999). In our experience the assay is a fast and reliable tool in the differential diagnosis of microangiopathic thrombocytopenia.

OC 08
Canthanox, a Randomised Controlled Study Comparing Low Molecular Weight Heparin and Warfarin for the Secondary Prevention of Venous Thromboembolism in Patients with Cancer

G MEYER, Z MARJANOVIC, J VALCKE, B LORCERIE, Y GRUEL, P SOLAL-CELIGNY, C LE MAIGNAN, JM EXTRA, P COTTU, D FARGE*
Service de pneumologie, hopital Europeen Georges Pompidou, Paris, France

The use of warfarin for treating venous thromboembolism in patients with cancer is associated with a significant risk of recurrence and bleeding. The use of low molecular weight heparin for secondary prevention of venous thromboembolism in cancer patients may reduce the complication rate. In a prospective randomised open–label multicentre trial, we compared subcutaneous enoxaparin (1.5 mg/kg once a day) with warfarin given for 3 months in 146 patients with venous thromboembolism and cancer. Diagnosis of deep-vein thrombosis was confirmed by venography or compression ultrasonography. Pulmonary embolism was confirmed by pulmonary angiography or ventilation/perfusion lung scanning indicating a high probability of pulmonary embolism, or a non-normal lung scan coinciding with objectively confirmed deep-vein thrombosis. Primary endpoint was a combined outcome event defined as major bleeding or recurrent venous thromboembolism within 3 months as judged by an independent adjudication committee, whose members were unaware of treatment assignment. Of the 71 evaluable patients assigned to receive warfarin, 15 (21.1%; 95% CI: 12.3-32.4%) experienced one major outcome event as compared to 7 of the 67 evaluable patients assigned to receive enoxaparin (10.5%; 95% CI: 4.3-20.3%; p=0.09). There were 6 deaths due to haemorrhage in the warfarin group as compared to none in the enoxaparin group. In the warfarin group, 17 patients died (22.7%; 95% CI: 13.8-33.8%) as compared to 8 in the enoxaparin group (11.3%; 95% CI: 5.0-21.0%; p=0.07). No difference was observed regarding the progression of the underlying cancer or cancer related death. These results confirm that warfarin is associated with a high failure rate in patients with venous thromboembolism and cancer. Prolonged treatment with low molecular weight heparin may be effective and safe in these patients.

OC 09
Lower Safety and Probably Lower Efficacy of Oral Anticoagulation (OA) in Cancer Patients with Venous Thromboembolism (VTE)

G PALARETI, C LEGNANI, B COSMI, S COCCHERI*
Dept. Angiology and Blood Coagulation,
University Hospital S. Orsola-Malpighi, Bologna, Italy

The optimal treatment of acute VTE in cancer patients remains undefined and controversial. Some studies, though not all, have reported a higher bleeding risk and more frequent VTE recurrences in patients with, than in those without, malignancy while on OA. Our study compared the outcome of anticoagulation courses in 95 patients with malignancy with those of 733 patients without malignancy. All patients were participants in a large, multicenter study and were prospectively followed from the initiation of their oral anticoagulant therapy. The quality of anticoagulation control was good: 70% of the time within the therapeutic range in both groups. Based on 744 patient-years of treatment and follow-up, the rates of major (5.4% vs 0.9%), minor (16.2% vs 3.6%) and total (21.6% vs 4.5%) bleeding were statistically significantly higher in cancer patients compared with patients without cancer. Bleeding was also a more frequent cause of early anticoagulation withdrawal in patients with malignancy (4.2% vs. 0.7%; p< 0.01; RR 6.2, 95% CI: 1.95-19.4). In the group of patients with cancer, the bleeding rate was high across the different INR categories and was independent of the temporally associated International Normalized Ratio (INR). In contrast, the bleeding rate was increased only with INR values greater than 4.5 in the group of patients without cancer. There was a trend towards a higher rate of thrombotic complications in cancer patients (6.8% vs. 2.5%; p=0.058; RR 2.5, 95% CI: 0.96-6.5) but this did not achieve statistical significance. The rate of thrombotic events was significantly higher in both cohorts when the INR was less than 2.0. Death was common in patients with cancer (31/95). The majority of deaths was secondary to the underlying cancer (90.3%), while only 6.5% of the deaths were attributed to PE in this patients group; however, it is possible that the real rate was higher because autopsies were not routinely performed. In conclusion, patients with malignancy treated with oral anticoagulants have a higher rate of bleeding and possibly an increased risk of recurrent thrombosis compared with patients without malignancy. Safer and more effective anticoagulant therapy is needed for this challenging group of patients.

OC 10
LMWH May Improve Long-Term Survival in Patients with Gastrointestinal Cancer

O THORLACIUS-USSING [1], LH IVERSEN [1], M OKHOLM [2], L PEDERSEN [3], H SØRENSEN [3]*
[1]Department of Surgical Gastroenterology, Aalborg Hospital and [2]Glostrup Hospital, and [3]Department of Clinical Epidemiology, University of Aarhus and Aalborg Hospital, Denmark

Background: Treatment studies of DVT have suggested LMWH to improve short-time survival in patients with metastatic cancer. However, no informations are available concerning long-term survival after prophylaxis with LMWH against postoperative thrombosis. **Aim:** We compared 5-year survival of patients, who underwent surgery for gastrointestinal cancer, assigned to receive either enoxaparin or unfractionated heparin as thrombo-prophylaxis. **Material & methods:** Two hundred patients undergoing surgery for suspected gastrointestinal cancer were assigned randomly and double-blind to thrombo-prophylaxis with enoxaparin 40 mg per day or unfractionated heparin 5000 IU three times per day for 7 to 12 days. Data on survival were obtained from the Danish Central Personal Registry. To summarize the survival of the patients over time we used the Kaplan-Meier analysis to construct survival curves, which then were compared with the results of the log-rank test. **Results:** Cancer was diagnosed in 184 of the 200 patients. Curative surgery was performed in 138 (78%) patients and was independent of the prophylaxis regime. DVT developed in 31 (18%), 11 patients in the enoxaparin-group and 20 in the heparin-group.

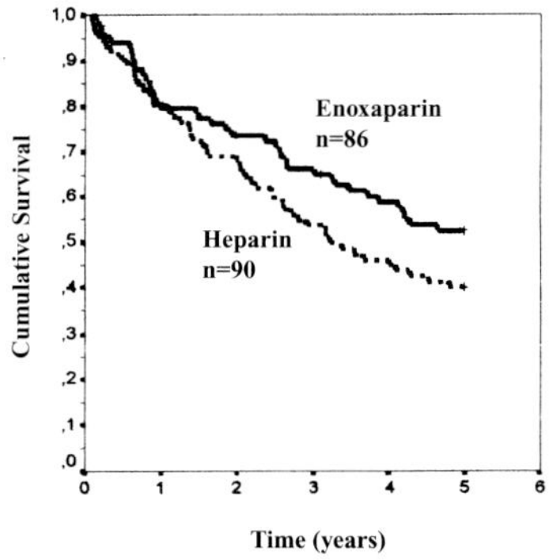

Overall 5-year survival in the enoxaparin-group (n=86) was 53% compared to 40% in the heparin-group (n=90), p=0.109. Excluding the patients, who had received oral anticoagulants due to postoperative DVT, these data were 52% in the LMWH-group (n=75) vs 42% in the heparin-group (n=70), p=0.231. A similar trend was observed analysing only patients who had curative surgery performed. **Conclusion:** Enoxaparin as thrombo-prophylaxis after surgery was associated with a non-significant improved 5-year survival compared to unfractionated heparin in patients with gastrointestinal cancer.

Hæmostasis

Poster Presentations

Haemostasis 2001;31(suppl. 1):78-107

PO 01

Do Inflammatory Adhesion Molecules and the Acute Phase Response Have a Role in Chemotherapy Induced Hypercoagulability?

CC KIRWAN, F TORELLA, CN MCCOLLUM, GJ BYRNE*
South Manchester University Hospital, Manchester, England

Introduction: Venous thromboembolism (VTE) is a recognised complication of cancer, particularly during chemotherapy. Chemotherapy-induced hypercoagulability may be stimulated through endothelial cell (EC) activation or an acute phase response. **Method:** Serum Vascular Cell Adhesion Molecule-1 (sVCAM-1), E-selectin (specific EC markers) and C-reactive protein (CRP) were measured before, and 1,3,5 and 7 days, and 3 months after chemotherapy in 11 patients with advanced and 14 patients with early breast or colorectal carcinoma. **Results:** Chemotherapy stimulated a significant and progressive fall in both E-selectin and sVCAM-1 over the first seven days from a median (IQR) of 40.3 (27.6-56.2) ng/ml and 416 (348-669) ng/ml respectively, before chemotherapy to 29.1 (25.1-45.8) ng/ml and 405 (346-585) ng/ml by day seven ($p<0.001$). CRP also had a significant decrease, from 4.7 (1-11.9) mg/l initially to only 2.8 (0.9-10.7) mg/l at day seven ($p=0.04$). E-selectin recovered to above pre-chemotherapy levels (47.1, 32.5-55.8 ng/ml) by three months as did sVCAM-1 (485, 377-552 ng/ml), but CRP remained low at only 1.6 (0.8-3.6) mg/l. Both E-selectin and sVCAM-1 were consistently higher with advanced cancer than with early cancer, but this was not statistically significant. There was a low-grade inflammatory response demonstrated by increased CRP at 9.0 (3.8-18.6) mg/l in advanced cancers, compared to only 1.59 (0.7-5.84) mg/l in early cancers ($p=0.05$). **Conclusions:** Plasma levels of E-selectin and sVCAM-1 fell progressively in the week following chemotherapy. This may be due to consumption of soluble forms of adhesion molecules by receptors on activated EC, reduced proteolysis of cell surface adhesion molecules, or competitive binding of soluble adhesion molecules to tumour cell fragments.

This alteration in EC activation may play a role in the chemotherapy-induced hypercoagulability of cancer. Hypercoagulability following chemotherapy does not appear to be due to an acute phase response.

PO 02

LMWH and UFH Counteract Endothelial Cell Tissue Factor (TF) Expression Induced by Breast Cancer Cell Media

A VIGNOLI, M MARCHETTI, T BARBUI, A FALANGA*
Hematology Division, Ospedali Riuniti, Bergamo, Italy

Heparin molecules are potent antithrombotics, which can exert multiple actions on the vessel wall. In this study we wanted to investigate whether heparins affect the procoagulant activity of vascular endothelial cells (EC) stimulated by tumor cells. Specifically, aims of the study were: 1. to characterize TF expression by human EC exposed to tumor cell conditioned media (CM) or to bacterial endotoxin (LPS) as a standard inflammatory stimulus; 2. to evaluate whether LMWH (dalteparin) and unfractionated heparin (UFH) are able to interfere with tumor cell CM- or LPS-induced endothelial TF. Human EC from both micro- (HMEC-1 line) and macro-vascular (HUVEC) beds were incubated for 4 h with CM from the human breast carcinoma cell line MDA-MB.231 (grown for 120 h) or LPS (10 μg/ml) or the vehicle (control) ± LMWH or UFH (from 0.01 to 10 IU/ml). After incubation, TF activity (TF:Act) was tested in EC lysates by the one-stage clotting assay, and TF antigen in EC extracts by ELISA. The results (mean ± SD of at least three experiments) show that the MDA-MB.231 CM significantly increased the expression of TF both in HMEC-1 and in HUVEC. The addition of the two heparins significantly affected this procoagulant expression. Specifically, in HMEC-1, 10 IU/ml dalteparin reduced TF expression induced by CM or LPS by 52±12% and 49±17%, respectively ($p<0.05$ vs controls), while UFH (10 IU/ml) by 39±8% and 41±15%, respectively ($p<0.05$ vs controls). There was a trend for dalteparin to be more effective than UFH in this condition. These results were confirmed by the analysis of TF antigen levels. In HUVEC, at the same concentration (10 IU/ml), dalteparin reduced the MDA-MB.231 CM- and LPS-induced TF:act by 53±15% and 27±8%, respectively, while UFH by 35±7% and 22±6%, respectively. In macrovascular EC dalteparin confirmed a trend to be more active than UFH on decreasing CM-induced TF, whereas both heparins showed to be less effective on LPS-induced TF in HUVEC compared to HMEC-1. These findings show that heparins can interfere with the local activation of coagulation triggered by tumor cell derived products or by LPS at the vascular site: a slight advantage for LMWH over UFH in the microvessel environment is suggested. Reducing TF expression by EC can contribute to reduce tumor neovascularization and disease progression.

PO 03
Tissue Factor Expression and Increased VEGF Secretion Proceed with Transition to Adherent Growth in a Small Cell Lung Cancer Cell Line

U SALGE, K BOLLER, E DAUBNER, M. HEIDEN, R SEITZ*
Paul-Ehrlich-Institut, Langen, Germany

Background: Tumor invasion and metastasis are thought to rely on cell adhesion and interaction with the vascular bed. Though small cell lung cancer (SCLC) clinically presents vigorous growth and formation of early metastases, cell lines in vitro, exhibit discrepant characteristics. They grow in suspension and only sparsely express proteolytic and procoagulant activity. The special complementary features of the selected adherent SCLC subline might delineate the potential of cells in vivo. **Methods:** The suspension SCLC line NCI-H69 was selected for adherent cells which were propagated separately. Growth parameters were determined in RPMI 1640 medium with 10% heat-inactivated FCS. Electron microscopy was performed on ultrathin sections of conventionally embedded cells. Expression of neural cell adhesion molecule (NCAM) and tissue factor (TF; monoclonal anti-TF, American Diagnostica) was determined by immunocytochemistry using the streptavidin-HRP Duett (DAKO) detection system. TF antigen was determined in cell homogenates and conditioned media by commercial ELISA (American Diagnostica). TF activity was measured colorimetrically via FXa generation. Secretion of vascular endothelial growth factor (VEGF) was determined by ELISA (ICN). **Results:** The suspension cell line SCLC NCI-H69 was selected for an adherent subline. These adherent cells still expressed NCAM, the histiotypic SCLC marker. Electron microscopy revealed fundamental morphological changes: expanded endoplasmic reticulum and formation of pseudopodia for adherent cells, alluding to increased protein synthesis and possible migratory capability. In contrast to parental suspension cells, adherent cells highly expressed functional TF which was paralleled by a five-fold increase in VEGF secretion. **Conclusion:** These observations describe the transition of a SCLC cell line from suspension to adherent growth. Concomitant changes of growth characteristics like morphology, induction of TF expression and increase in VEGF secretion may indicate the potential to express features believed to be essential for invasion and metastasis and might provide a model for the study of mechanisms involved in SCLC metastasis.
(Supported by Deutsche Krebshilfe, grant 70-2117-Se3)

PO 04
Apoptosis Induced by All-Trans Retinoic Acid (ATRA) is Associated with a Reduction of Procoagulant Activity (PCA) in Human Breast Cancer Cells

M MARCHETTI, D BALDUCCI, S SUARDI, T BARBUI, A FALANGA*
Hematology Division, Ospedali Riuniti, Bergamo, Italy

Drug-induced cellular apoptosis is associated with an increased expression of PCA by malignant cells, which may contribute to the thrombogenicity of anti-tumor therapies. Differently, in human promyelocytic leukemia cells, apoptosis induced by ATRA is associated with down regulation of tumor cell PCA, i.e. Tissue Factor (TF) and Cancer Procoagulant (CP). It is known that ATRA exerts anti-proliferative and pro-apoptotic effects on human breast cancer cells, however its action on the PCA of these cells is yet unknown. We have analysed different human breast cancer cell lines in order to: 1. characterize the modulation of TF and CP by ATRA; 2. verify the relationship of ATRA-induced modification of tumor cell procoagulants with the apoptotic effects of this agent. Two estrogen receptor positive (ER+; MCF-7 and ZR-75-1) and one ER negative (ER-; MDA-MB-231) breast cancer cell lines, with low and high metastatic potential, respectively, were studied. The results show that all the three cell types express both TF and CP. Maximum TF and CP levels were found in the highly metastasizing MDA-MB-231 cells.

After 96 h incubation with ATRA, TF and CP expression were significantly reduced in all the three cell lines. At the same time, in the two ER+ cell lines, a significant inhibition of cell proliferation by ATRA was detected by the analysis of growth curves. This phenomenon was associated with a significant induction of apoptosis, as demonstrated by the increase in the percentage of Annexin V-positive cells and decrease in Bcl-2 oncoprotein levels. A slight inhibition of cell proliferation with virtually no signs of apoptosis occurred in the ER- MDA-MB.231 cell line treated with ATRA. This study shows that ATRA downregulates the expression of TF and CP in breast cancer cells. In ER+ cells this effect occurs concomitantly to apoptosis and cell growth inhibition induced by the drug, suggesting that ATRA counteracts the procoagulant effect associated to apoptotic phenomena in solid tumor cells. We speculate that ATRA in combination with chemotherapy may protect against the procoagulant stimulus of cytotoxic drugs on malignant cells. (Supported by the Italian Association for Cancer Research, AIRC).

PO 05
Effects of 9-cis Retinoic Acid (9-Cis RA) on the Procoagulant Activity (PCA) of Breast Cancer Cells

D BALDUCCI, M MARCHETTI, S SUARDI, T BARBUI, A FALANGA*
Hematology Division, Ospedali Riuniti, Bergamo, Italy.

All-trans retinoic acid (ATRA) inhibits proliferation and induces apoptosis in breast cancer cells. In addition ATRA reduces the PCA (i. e., tissue factor, TF; and cancer procoagulant, CP) of these cells. In other solid tumor cells, the isomer 9-cis RA, a retinoic acid (RARs) and retinoic X receptors (RXRs) pan-agonist, is more effective than ATRA (selective RARs agonist), on cell growth and apoptosis; its effect on PCA is yet unknown. In this study, we investigated whether 9-cis RA can modulate TF and CP in parallel with its effects on growth and apoptosis of breast cancer cells and the results were compared with those induced by ATRA. Two estrogen receptor positive (ER+; i.e. MCF-7 and ZR-75-1) and one ER negative (ER-; i.e. MDA-MB-231) breast cancer cell lines were incubated with retinoids (10-6M) for 96h and tested for PCA, apoptosis and cell growth. The results on TF show that: 1. in MCF-7 cells, 9-cis RA significantly reduced TF expression, but less effectively than ATRA (19% vs 42% inhibition, $p<0.05$); 2. in ZR-75-1 cells, both retinoids had equal activity on TF inhibition; and, 3. in MDA-MB-231 cells, 9-cis RA had virtually no effects on TF, whereas ATRA reduced TF by 28%. Concerning CP expression, both retinoids significantly reduced CP in all the cell lines, ATRA being always more effective than 9-cis RA ($p<0.05$). In the two ER+ cell lines, ATRA and 9-cis RA induced apoptosis to the same extent; in addition, ATRA was more effective than 9-cis RA on cell proliferation inhibition (ATRA versus 9-cis RA: $p<0.05$). In MDA-MB-231 cells virtually no apoptosis occurred with either ATRA or 9-cis RA. These results indicate that 9-cis RA is capable but less effective than ATRA in downregulating TF and CP of breast cancer cells, suggesting a minor role of RXRs in modulating cellular procoagulants. In ER+ cells TF and CP reduction by 9-cis RA is associated with a lower effect on cell growth inhibition and apoptosis. Therefore 9-cis RA appears less potent than ATRA on both proliferation and PCA modulation in breast cancer cells. (Supported by the Italian Association for Cancer Research, AIRC).

PO 06
Procoagulant Activity of Four T-Lymphoblastoid Cell Lines: Role of Tissue Factor, Phospholipid and Cancer Procoagulant

W PICKERING[1], E GRAY[1], AH GOODALL[2], TW BARROWCLIFFE[1]*
[1]NIBSC, Potters Bar, and [2]Division of Chemical Pathology Leicester University, UK.

It is well established that monocytes can exhibit procoagulant activity (PCA), mainly due to tissue factor (TF), however less is known about lymphocyte PCA. This study was designed to evaluate the levels of phospholipid (PL) like TF-independent PCA, TF activity and the influence of Cancer Procoagulant (CP), in T-Lymphoblastoid cell lines. Four T-cell lines CCRF-CEM, JURKAT, MOLT 4 and A3.01, as well as a control Monocytoid cell line THP-1, were cultured under standard conditions washed in RPMI, and suspended in Tris buffer. All cells used were >90% viable. TF activity was measured by shortening of buffer clotting times of platelet poor plasma (PPP). The time course of PL-dependent FXa generation was measured by incubating human FX, FIXa, FVIII with cells or different concentrations of PL and CaCl2. This system was modified to detect CP by omitting FIXa, FVIII from the system. TF activity and PL-dependent Xa generation was found in all cell lines studied. CP was not responsible for the Xa generation observed. The results are shown in the table below.
These results confirm that certain T-Lymphoid cell lines show TF-independent PCA by acting as active surfaces for the "tenase" complex. The relative activity of the four cell lines is not related to their TF activity but appears to be higher in the more differentiated cells. This finding may have some relevance as a contributory factor for the atypical finding of thrombosis in some ALL patients.

PO 07
Is Hyperfibrinogenemia in Patients with Small Cell Carcinoma of the Lung Inflammatory Response to Tumor Cells?

T WAJIMA, DD VON HOFF*
Texas A&M University and Central Texas Veterans Health Care System, Temple, Texas and University of Texas Health Science Center at San Antonio, Texas, USA

Background: Hyperfibrinogenemia is a common finding in patients with small cell carcinoma of the lung (SCCL), and is also reversible when complete remission is achieved by systemic chemotherapy. Plasma fibrinogen is an acute phase-reacting protein. Inflammatory cells such as macrophage/monocyte, T-lymphocyte, and endothelial cells secrete IL-6, IL-1 & TNF that induce acute phase-reacting response. Plasma fibrinogen is produced only by the hepatic cells through IL-6. Plasma fibrinogen levels tend to correlate with circulating IL-6, not with IL-1 or TNF. We investigated the secretion of IL-6, IL-1, and TNF

Table to abstract P0-06:

Cell Line Conc 4x10^6	TF Activity Arbitrary TF Units. Mean and 95% CI	CP Activity	PL-dependent FXa Activity Arbitrary PL Units. Mean and 95% CI
CCRF-CEM	0.22 0.183 – 0.256	Not Detected	14 13 - 17
JURKAT	0.513 0.432 – 0.594	Not Detected	18 16 - 20
MOLT 4	0.051 0.044 – 0.059	Not Detected	34 29 - 40
A3.01	0.038 0.032 – 0.044	Not Detected	40 35 - 46
THP-1	1.777 1.501 – 2.054	Not Detected	12 10 - 14

by SCCL tumor cells in the presence of hyperfibrinogenemia. **Material & Methods:** Twenty patients with SCCL were studied. Single cell suspensions of SCCL were processed according to the stem cell assay technique. The supernatant of single cell suspension was made. The levels of IL-6, IL-1, & TNF in plasma and extract of single cell suspension were measured by ELISA. Plasma fibrinogen was assayed by routine clotting method.
Results: In the extract of single cell suspension IL-6, IL-1 and TNF were not detected by this method. Plasma IL-6 levels were higher than control. Plasma IL-1 and TNF were within normal limits. Plasma fibrinogen levels were increased in all patients. **Limitation:** Single cell suspensions (tumor cell alone) are different from tumor tissue (the tumor tissue consists of tumor cells and stroma cells such as macrophage, fibroblast or endothelial cell). These stroma cells secrete cytokines. **Conclusions:** Tumor cells of SCCL do not secrete detectable levels of IL-6. Elevated levels of IL-6 derive from macrophage/ monocyte, T-lymphocyte, and endothelial cells rather than tumor cells.

PO 08
Sensitivity to Anti-Angiogenic Compounds of Endothelial Cells Derived from Human Tumors and Normal Tissues

R DOSSI [1], MR BANI [1], G ALESSANDRI [2], G TARABOLETTI [1], R GIAVAZZI [1]*
[1]Laboratory of Biology and Treatment of Metastasis, Mario Negri Institute for Pharmacological Research, Bergamo; [2]Institute of Microbiology University of Brescia, Italy

Endothelial cells present a tissue-specific phenotypic heterogeneity, acquired in response to micro-environmental stimuli. There is evidence that tumour-associated endothelial cells differ from endothelial cells of normal tissues. Since anti-angiogenic therapies aimed at blocking the formation of new vessels in tumours are currently proposed as antineoplastic agents, in this study we examined the response of tumour-derived endothelial cells to anti-angiogenic compounds. To this purpose, we have isolated endothelial cells from different tissues (umbilical vein, adrenal gland, derma, kidney and ovarian and renal carcinomas). Expression of von Willebrand Factor (vWF) and CD31, and lack of positivity for alpha-Smooth Muscle Actin confirmed the purity of the preparations. The proliferative stimuli – e.g. VEGF, bFGF, EGF - have demonstrated to be powerful inducers of proliferation for all the types of endothelium. However, a higher percentage of tumour-derived endothelial cells expressed SA-beta-galactosidase (a marker for senescent cells), compared to endothelial cells isolated from normal tissues. Such a premature senescent phenotype correlated with the early loss of responsiveness to proliferative stimuli. The sensitivity of the different endothelial cells to three compounds that inhibit angiogenesis with different mechanisms of action was investigated: TNP-470 (an antiproliferative agent), SU5416 (a VEGFR antagonist) and paclitaxel (a tubulin binding drug). All the compounds inhibited the proliferation of endothelial cells. We have seen no difference in response between endothelial cells isolated from tumours and normal tissues. No differences were also observed among the different tumor-derived endothelial cell preparations. Similarly, paclitaxel also inhibited migration of the endothelium of various origin. Tumour-derived endothelial cells cultured in vitro can be a useful tool to study the effectiveness of angiogenesis inhibitors. In the same experimental conditions, the sensitivity to anti-angiogenic compounds was similar to that of endothelium isolated from normal tissues. Endothelial cells from tumours, in vitro, lost quickly their replicative ability and acquired a premature senescent phenotype compared to the endothelial cells from normal tissues.

PO 09
The Tumor Microenvironment Modulates Endothelial Cells Gene Expression: Identification of a Differentially Expressed Transcript

*C GHILARDI[1] *, R DOSSI[1], G ALESSANDRI[2], MR BANI[1], R GIAVAZZI[1]*
[1]Laboratory of the Biology and Treatment of Metastasis, M. Negri Institute, Bergamo; [2]Institute of Microbiology, University of Brescia, Italy

Solid tumors are able to promote the formation of new blood vessels from which they depend for their growth and metastatization. During the angiogenesis process, quiescent endothelial cells undergo molecular, morphological and functional changes. To understand how the tumor microenvironment influences gene expression in endothelial cells, HAMEC (Human Adrenal Microvascular Endothelial cells) were placed under in vitro "tumor/angiogenesis"-related environment. This consisted of oncofetal fibronectin and cancer-released angiogenic factors, which we have found to be the optimum conditions for the growth and proliferation of tumor-derived endothelial cells (Clin Exp Met 1999;17:655-662). Then, we compared the genotype expression of exposed and unexposed HAMEC by virtue of Differential Display. As expected, expression patterns of the two populations were mostly identical. However, we were able to identify a differentially expressed transcript of 1.1 Kb. Northern Blot analysis showed that its expression was downregulated when endothelial cells, both HAMEC and HUVEC, were placed under in vitro "tumor/angiogenesis"-related environment. In contrast, no modulation was achieved when different types of tumor cells (i.e. melanoma and ovarian, kidney and colon carcinoma cells) were analyzed. In addition to tumor-derived fibronectin, other matrix proteins, involved in remodeling of the extracellular matrix during angiogenesis, modulated its expression in endothelial cells. No changes in the level of expression of the transcript were observed when endothelial cells were placed under hypoxic condition. The analysis of the sequence obtained so far showed that the gene product is a protein, comprising four trans-membrane domains. (Supported by the Italian Association for Cancer Research , A.I.R.C.)

PO 10
Tissue Factor-Mediated Induction of Capillary Formation In Vitro

*C ETTELAIE [1], NJ JAMES [2] *, K RICHARD BRUCKDORFER [1]*
[1]Biomedical Section, Dept. of Biological Science, University of Hull, Hull and [2]Dept. of Biochemistry and Molecular Biology, RF&UCMS, London, UK

Tissue factor (TF) is a cell surface receptor that is expressed upon injury or trauma and is principal initiator of coagulation. Moreover, the regulatory role of TF in the proliferation of vascular cells has been acknowledged [1]. Recent literature suggests different mechanisms for the cellular-receptor function of the tissue factor [2]. These include pathways mediated via activated coagulation factors VIIa and Xa, for example, by subsequent digestion of PAR-1 and PAR-2 [3] and the intracellular domain of TF [4]. The effect is to modulate blood vessel formation [1]. Our preliminary data suggest that while tissue factor itself may induce vascularisation, its interaction with blood proteases, factor VII and X can lead to induction of vessel regression. In experiments using a collagen gel model for angiogenesis, it was found that addition of exogenous tissue factor to the cells accelerated microvessel formation to an extent similar to that of the positive control (2 μM VEGF). In contrast, the inclusion of serum proteases factor VII and X in the presence of tissue factor inhibited the angiogenesis, to a level below that of untreated cultures (5 μM suramin). Furthermore, a reduction in the number of viable cells was observed in these test samples. The support of The Royal Society and the Yorkshire Cancer Research is acknowledged.

1. Chen, J. et al Thromb .Haemostas. 86, 334-345 (2001)
2. Ruf, W., Mueller, BM. Thromb. Haemostas. 82, 175-182 (1999)
3. Camerer, E. et al Proc. Natl. Acad. Sci. USA 97, 5255-5260 (2000)
4. Abe, K., et al. Proc. Natl. Acad. Sci. USA 96, 8663-8668 (1999)

PO 11
Thrombospondin-1 Modulates Angiogenic Factors Interaction with the Extracellular Matrix: A Potential Mechanism of Tsp-1 Antiangiogenic Activity

B MARGOSIO, V VERGANI, P BORSOTTI, R GIAVAZZI, G TARABOLETTI*
Laboratory of Biology and Treatment of Metastasis, Dept. Oncology, Mario Negri Institute for Pharmacological Research, Bergamo, Italy

The antiangiogenic molecule thrombospondin-1 (TSP-1) binds with high affinity to several angiogenic factors, including FGF-2 (bFGF), VEGF and HGF/SF. In this study we have investigated the functional consequences of TSP-1 binding to these growth factors. We previously reported that TSP-1 prevents the binding of FGF-2 to its low affinity receptors (heparansulfate proteoglycans, HSPGs) on endothelial cells, and reduces the internalization of the growth factor. These findings suggest that TSP-1 might affect the interaction of the angiogenic factors with the HSPGs in the extracellular matrix (ECM), an important mechanism of regulation of location, availability and activity of the heparin-binding angiogenic factors. Here we show that TSP-1 dose-dependently prevented the binding of labelled FGF-2 to the ECM, up to a degree comparable with heparin. Binding of labelled FGF-2 to the ECM was not affected by preincubation of the matrix with TSP-1, suggesting that the mechanism of inhibition was not due to the competition between FGF-2 and TSP-1 for the binding to HSPGs in the matrix. TSP-1 also dose-dependently caused the release of ECM-associated FGF-2. Crosslinking and immuno-precipitation experiments demonstrated that FGF-2 was released by TSP-1 as a complex FGF-2/TSP-1. FGF-2 released from the matrix by TSP-1 was not able to induce endothelial cells proliferation. The region of TSP-1 responsible for both the inhibition of binding and the release of FGF-2 from the matrix was located within the 140 kDa, antiangiogenic fragment of the molecule, which contains the binding site for FGF-2. TSP-1 also inhibited VEGF and HGF/SF binding to the ECM and caused their release when they were ECM-associated. Our study shows that TSP-1 regulates the interaction of angiogenic factors with the ECM, therefore affecting their availability and activity. This could represent an additional mechanism of the antiangiogenic activity of TSP-1. (Supported by the Italian Association for Cancer Research, A.I.R.C.)

PO 12
The Interaction between Endothelial and Myeloma Cells and the Effects of Verotoxin

G MOLOSTVOV, A MORRIS, P ROSE, S BASU*
Department of Biological Sciences, University of Warwick, Coventry; Department of Haematology, Warwick Hospital, Warwick, UK

We studied CD77 expression and verotoxin (VT) induced apoptosis in human umbilical vein endothelial cells (HUVEC) and myeloma cells separately and in co-culture. As a myeloma model system, we used parental line RPMI-8226/S (drug-sensitive) and its drug-resistant variants - Dox 40 (doxorubicin-resistant) and LR5 (melphalan-resistant). CD77 expression was measured by flow cytometry using specific monoclonal antibody (Coulter) while apoptosis was detected using annexin V and propidium iodide staining (Calbiochem). We revealed that unstimulated HUVEC had very low expression of CD77 and were resistant to apoptosis induced by VT. CD77 level in RPMI-8226/S and its variants varied from 30-40% (+) in Dox 40 and LR5 to 60-70% (++) in 8226/S line. Interestingly, our experiments showed that drug-resistant lines were also less sensitive to the apoptotic action of VT (10 ng/ml for up to 48 hours). Interaction between myeloma cells and endothelium is thought to be of crucial importance for myeloma cell survival and growth. Co-culture experiments revealed various degrees of adhesion with myeloma/endothelium cell adhesion ratio ranging from 1/9 in LR5 to 2/1 in 8226/S as soon as after 2 hours of co-culturing. From experiments with VT-induced cell death we found that the levels of apoptosis in 8226/S and Dox 40 were significantly (p from 0.01 to 0.05) lower in co-culture than in myeloma cells cultured without HUVEC both at 6 and 24 hours of VT treatment. Basal levels of apoptosis in myeloma cells were also significantly lower in co-culture compared to the cells cultured alone. Our data suggest that myeloma/endothelial cells interactions in co-culture have a significant protective effect on both basal and VT-induced levels of apoptosis in myeloma cells.

PO 13
Expression of VEGF, MMP2 & MMP9 in Plasma and Ascites of Patients Affected by Ovarian Carcinoma

P PAGANONI[1]*, L MANENTI[1], I FLORIANI[2], G TARABOLETTI[1], F LANDONI[3], D BELOTTI[1], R GIAVAZZI[1]
[1]Laboratory of Biology and Treatment of Metastasis, Mario Negri Institute for Pharmacological Research, Bergamo; [2]Laboratory Oncological Clinical Reserch, Mario Negri Institute for Pharmacological Research, Milan; [3]Department of Obstetrics and Gynecology , S. Gerardo Hospital, Monza, Italy

Vascular Endothelial Growth Factor (VEGF) and Matrix Metalloproteases (MMPs) are highly expressed in human malignancies and are believed to play a pivotal role in tumor angiogenesis, growth and metastasis. In this study, we have measured the levels of the angiogenic factor VEGF and MMP9 & MMP2 in plasma of patients affected by ovarian carcinoma (n=42), patients affected by non-neoplastic gynecological pathologies (n=28) and in plasma of healthy volunteers (n=26). The levels of MMPs (pro and active forms) were measured by zymography and quantified by image analyze. The levels of soluble VEGF were determined by ELISA technique. Preoperative plasma VEGF levels in patients affected by ovarian carcinomas were significantly higher than in healthy volunteers and in patients affected by non-neoplastic gynecological pathologies. Also, high levels of proMMP9 and proMMP2 were detected in plasma of patients affected by ovarian carcinoma; significally high levels of activated MMP9 were found. Since ovarian cancer is characterized by widespread intraperitoneal tumors and formation of ascitic fluid, we also studied the levels of VEGF and MMPs in ascitic fluids of the patients with ovarian carcinoma. Elevated levels of both factors were found. To further analyze the relationship between MMPs and VEGF in biological fluids, xenograft models of human ovarian carcinoma transplanted in the peritoneal cavity of nude mice were used. Accordingly, MMP2 & MMP9 and VEGF were present at higher levels in ascites of mice bearing tumors than in peritoneal washes of healthy ones. The levels of MMPs and VEGF in ascites correlated with the tumor burden. In conclusion, we have found that high levels of VEGF and MMPs in biological fluids were related to the presence of ovarian malignancy and associated with disease progression.

PO 14
Pai-1 is a Molecular Target for Hyperthermia-Mediated Inhibition of Angiogenesis

C ROCA[1]*, L PRIMO[1], D VALDEMBRI[1], P GABRIELE[2], P CARMELIET[3], A CIVIDALLI[4], F BUSSOLINO[1,5]
[1]Division of Molecular Angiogenesis, Institute for Cancer Research and Treatment, Candiolo, Italy; [2]Division of Radiotherapy, Mauriziano Hospital, Torino, Italy; [3]The Center for Transgene Technology and Gene Therapy, Flanders Interuniversity Institute for Biotechnology, Leuven, Belgium; [4]Divisione di Medicina e Biomedicina, ENEA CR Casaccia, Rome, Italy; [5]Department of Genetics, Biology and Biochemistry, University of Torino, Italy

Hyperthermia combined with radiotherapy or chemotherapy is a promising method for cancer treatment. The mechanisms of how hyperthermia inhibits tumor growth are not well understood. We evaluated the hyperthermia treatment on angiogenesis, the process of development of new vessels from pre-existing ones. We studied the hyperthermia effects on the capillary-like structures formation in three-dimensional culture system, consisting of extracellular matrix protein. In Matrigel model, endothelial cells with appropriate stimulus (VEGF, bFGF) make capillary-like structures, in a process named "in vitro angiogenesis". Hyperthermia treatment affected these structures, blocking the tubular morphogenesis induced by vascular endothelial growth factor (VEGF). Hyperthermia also affected the ability of human endothelial (EC) cells to sprout in response to appropriate stimuli in collagen spheroid model. To confirm our in vitro data, we used the chicken embryo chorioallantoic membrane assay, a well-established in vivo angiogenesis model. In our study, after stimulation with 20 ng/ml VEGF-A and treatment at 43 °C for 1 hour, we observed the completely inhibition of new vessels formation. In the same experimental conditions, cultured human EC, did not show a decreased viability, suggesting that the reduced angiogenic activity was not due to heat induced cytotoxicity. By analysing hyperthermia treated EC on DNA microarray, we defined a pattern of gene expression that correlates with the lost ability to produce new vessels. In particular, we showed enhanced expression of two genes involved in process of extracellular matrix degradation: TIMP-1 (tissue inhibitor of metalloproteinase-1) and PAI-1 (human plasminogen activator inhibitor-1). This pattern of expression could explain the behaviour of endothelial cells after hyperthermia treatment in angiogenesis assays. To confirm the central role of PAI-1 in angiogenesis inhibition by hyperthermia treatment, we analyzed the behaviour of EC on Matrigel in the presence of neutralizing antibody anti-PAI-1. The addition of anti-PAI-1 antibody reverted heat-induced inhibition of vessel formation on Matrigel assay. Moreover, we evaluated the expression level of PAI-1 in a murine tumor model (the TSA mammary adenocarcinoma) and observed an increased level of PAI-1 in tumors heated for 1 h at 43 °C. Hyperthermia affects also the tumor vasculature: by using an anti-FVIII antibody, that specifically stains EC, we observed a drastic reduction of vascularization and consequently a large area of necrosis. Our data underline the biological role of heat treatment in the inhibition of angiogenesis and suggest that new vessel formation could be the target of hyperthermia.

PO 15
Combination of Chemotherapy and Anticoagulant Drugs for the Treatment of Malignant Tumors

VA SUKHANOV, LP MALCHIKOVA, LD GERASIMOVA*
Haemostas. Lab., Regional Hospital NI, Ekaterinsburg, Russia

Myelosuppression is known to limit the ability of patients to take maximally effective cytotoxic therapy. Thrombosis of vessels supplying tumor is probably one of the main reasons for it. The aim of the study was to combine chemotherapy and anticoagulants to avoid myelosuppression and to make cytotoxic therapy more effective. Fifty-eight patients (pts) with different malignant tumors of the head were considered for this study. The first 28 pts were treated with cytotoxic drugs without anticoagulants (control group). The next 30 pts (investigated group) received chemotherapy in combination with anticoagulant drugs (Low Molecular Weight Heparin-Fraxiparine, 0.3 ml daily during the first 10-14 days plus Warfarin during 2-2.5 years, therapeutic range: INR = 1.5-2.0). During the treatment period pts of the two groups were identical in dose of cytotoxic drugs per time unit, morphology of tumor and its localization. The study demonstrated that there was myelosuppression in 2 pts (7%) of control group that necessitated withdrawal of chemotherapy untimely. Another 3 pts (11%) of this group had relapse of the illness during 2 years of follow up. In the investigated group of pts taking anticoagulants there were no complications of chemotherapy. Moreover, we noticed that on the 4-8th day of chemotherapy there was increase of leycocyte count in peripheral blood from $4.8x10^9/L$ + $0.7x10^9/L$ (mean±SD) to $7.2x10^9/L±1.4x10^9/L$, p = 0.05. Only 5 pts (17%) had some decrease of leycocyte count to $4.1x10^9/L± 0.3x10^9/L$ (p>0.05) at the end of chemotherapy treatment. In the follow up period (from 2 to 4 years) there was neither relapse of the illness nor metastasis. In summary, combination of chemotherapy with anticoagulation increases efficiency of treatment of malignant tumors and decreases the complications of cytotoxic drugs.

PO 16
Anti-Angiogenic Efficacy & Mechanism of the Low Molecular Weight Heparin, Tinzaparin and Tissue Factor Pathway Inhibitor: Anti-Cancer Benefits

*SA MOUSA**
DuPont Pharmaceuticals Co., Wilmington, DE, USA

Background: Initial clinical trials have indicated a significant effect of LMWH, as compared to UFH on the survival of cancer patients with deep vein thrombosis. Hence, the present study was undertaken to define the role and mechanism of the LMWH Tinzaparin on the modulation of angiogenesis. **Methods:** The effects of the LMWH contributing components such as the anti-Xa, anti-IIa and TFPI on the modulation of angiogenesis related processes including in vitro endothelial tube formation and in vivo angiogenesis-mediated by angiogenic factors and cancer cells were studied. The in vivo effects of Innhohep and r-TFPI on angiogenesis were studied in the chick chorioallantoic membrane (CAM) model. Twenty-four hours after stimulating angiogenesis with basic fibroblast growth factor (FGF2), vascular endothelial growth factor, tissue factor (TF), lipopolysaccharide (LPS) or colon and lung carcinoma, test agents were directly applied to the growth factor saturated filter disk or injected intravenously into the embryonic circulation. **Results:** Data demonstrated significant and comparable inhibitory effects of Tinzaparin or r-TFPI in a concentration-dependent manner on endothelial cell tube formation. Both Tinzaparin and r-TFPI blocked FGF2, VEGF, other angiogenic factors, TF and LPS-induced angiogenesis in the CAM model by 80-100%. Additionally, a significant inhibition of colon lung carcinoma growth and regression occurred after treatment with Tinzaparin or r-TFPI. Furthermore, the anti-angiogenesis efficacy in relation to endothelial cell TFPI release for different heparin molecular weight fractions within Tinzaparin was examined. Heparin fractions with molecular weight closer to 3,000 Dalton was shown to be ineffective both in releasing endothelial cell TFPI and in inhibiting angiogenesis as compared to a very effective heparin fractions with molecular weight ranging from 5,000-8,000 Dalton. Both Tinzaparin and r-TFPI promoted EC apoptosis (P53 and DNA fragmentation). The anti-angiogenesis-mediated effects of Tinzaparin were blocked by a specific TFPI monoclonal antibody, with TF/VIIa binding domain but not anti-TFPI with Xa binding domain. **Conclusions:** These studies demonstrated a significant role for Tinzaparin and its in vivo releasable TFPI on the regulation of angiogenesis and tumor growth. Thus, Tinzaparin might be a useful therapeutic for the inhibition of angiogenesis associated with human tumor growth, atherosclerotic and inflammatory desease.

PO 17
Anti-Metastatic Effect of Low Molecular Weight Heparin Tinzaparin and Tissue Factor Pathway Inhibitor

*A AMIRKHOSRAVI, J FRANCIS, S MOUSA**
Walt Disney Memorial Cancer Institute at Florida Hospital Orlando, FL, and Dupont Pharmaceuticals Company, Wilmington, DE, USA

The significance of Tissue factor (TF) in cancer biology is suggested by studies reporting its involvement in metastasis and angiogenesis. Tinzaparin is a low molecular weight heparin (LMWH) that is produced by heparinase depolymerization of unfractionated heparin allowing for its relatively high sulfate to carboxylate ratio. Beyond its potent plasmatic effects on ATIII-dependent coagulation factors, Tinzaparin is a very effective LMWH in causing the release of TFPI from the endothelial cells, the natural inhibitor of tissue factor procoagulant and non-coagulant effects. The present study was undertaken to investigate the effect of the LMWH, Tinzaparin as well as recombinant TFPI on experimental lung metastasis. Using the B16 melanoma injectable model of metastasis, we found that subcutaneous injection of Tinzaparin (10 mg/kg) 4 hrs before intravenous injection of 2.5 x 10^5 melanoma cells, reduced lung tumor formation in experimental mice by 89% (31±23 vs 3±2, p<0.001). In a second experimental group, in addition to the initial (pre-tumor cell) dose, subcutaneous Tinzaparin (10 mg/kg) was administered daily for 14 days at which time lung seeding was assessed. In the latter group, lung tumor formation was reduced by 96% (p<0.001). No bleeding problems were observed in any of the heparinized animals. In order to determine the anticoagulant activity of Tinzaparin, 4 hrs after a single subcutaneous dose, whole blood recalcification was measured using a Sonoclot Analyzer. Tinzaparin (10 mg/kg S.C.) prolonged the clotting time 4-fold. Furthermore, the effect of Tinzaparin on tumor cell- induced clotting activation in vivo was determined by measuring the platelet count (a sensitive marker of intravascular coagulation) before and 15 minutes after tumor cell injection in control and Tinzaparin-treated animals. Following i.v. injection of 2 x 10^6 tumor cells, a rapid and significant fall in platelet count was observed (from 939±37 x 10^6/ml to 498±94 x 10^6 /ml, p<0.001). In Tinzaparin-treated animals, a significant reversal to normal platelet count was achieved (921±104 x 10^6/ml). Intravenous injection of TFPI (700 ng) 5 minutes prior to tumor cell injection, also reduced B16 lung metastasis (85%, p<0.01) and abolished tumor cell induced thrombocytopenia. Our results support the potential role of the LMWH Tinzaparin and its reseasable TFPI in tumor metastasis.

PO 18
Anticoagulant in Thrombosis & Cancer: The Missing Link

*S MOUSA**
DuPont Pharmaceuticals Co, Wilmington DE, USA

Many cancer patients reportedly have hypercoagulable state, with recurrent thrombosis due to the impact of cancer cells and chemotherapy on the coagulation cascade. Studies have demonstrated that UFH or its low molecular weight fractions interfere with various processes involved in tumor growth and metastasis. These include fibrin formation, binding of heparin to angiogenic growth factors such as basic fibroblast growth factor (FGF2) and VEGF, modulation of tissue factor, and perhaps other modulatory mechanisms. Clinical trials have indicated a clinically relevant effect of low molecular weight heparin (LMWH), as compared to unfractionated heparin (UFH) on the survival of cancer patients with deep vein thrombosis. Similarly, the impact of Warfarin (Coumadin) on the survival of cancer patients with thromboembolic disorders was demonstrated. Hence, the present study was undertaken to define the role of the LMWH (Tinzaparin), Coumadin, anti-factor VIIa and recombinant tissue factor pathway inhibitor (r-TFPI) on the modulation of angiogenesis. The effects of Tinzaparin, Coumadin, anti-VIIa and r-TFPI on the modulation of angiogenesis related processes including in vitro endothelial tube formation and in vivo angiogenesis-mediated by angiogenic factors and cancer cells were studied. The in vivo effects of those different anticoagulants on angiogenesis were studied in the chick chorioallantoic membrane (CAM) model. Twenty-four hours after stimulating angiogenesis on the CAM with FGF2, lipopolysaccharide (LPS) or colon carcinoma (HCT-116), Tinzaparin, Coumadin, anti-VIIa or r-TFPI were directly applied to the growth factor saturated filter disk or were injected intravenously into the embryonic circulation. Data demonstrated significant and comparable inhibitory effect of Tinzaparin, anti-VIIa or r-TFPI in a concentration-dependent manner on endothelial cell tube formation. Both Tinzaparin, Coumadin, anti-VIIa and r-TFPI blocked FGF2-induced angiogenesis in the CAM model by 80-100%. Additionally, a significant inhibition of colon carcinoma growth and regression was demonstrated with Tinzaparin, Coumadin, Anti-VIIa and r-TFPI. These studies demonstrated a significant role for Tinzaparin, Coumadin, anti-VIIa and Tinzaparin releasable TFPI on the regulation of angiogenesis and tumor growth. Thus, modulation of tissue factor / VIIa non-coagulant activities by Tinzaparin, Coumadin, anti-VIIa or TFPI might be a useful therapeutic for the inhibition of angiogenesis associated with human tumor growth, neovascular related ocular and inflammatory diseases.

PO 19
The Risk of a Venous Thrombotic Event in Lung Cancer Patients

JW BLOM, S OSANTO, FR ROSENDAAL*
Leiden University Medical Center, Department of Clinical Epidemiology, Leiden, Netherlands

The association between cancer and venous thrombotic events (VTE) has been recognised since 1868 (Trousseau), but only limited data on the incidence of VTE in different types of malignancy are available. Thrombosis and cancer are clearly related: 7.3% of patients with idiopathic thrombosis develop malignancy compared to 1.6% of patients with thrombosis occurring in the presence of known risk factors (Hettiarachchi, Cancer 1998;83:180-5). Patients with adenocarcinoma are believed to have the highest risk of developing a VTE during the course of their disease. Among malignancies presenting with venous thromboembolism as a first clinical manifestation, prostate and colorectal cancer are the most commonly identified. Also cancers of the pancreas, stomach, lung and ovary are frequently identified. To study the incidence of thrombosis in various types of cancer, with an emphasis on the comparison between different histological types of cancer, we have initiated an ongoing cohort study of patients with non small cell lung cancer. A total of 318 patients who had their initial diagnosis of lung carcinoma in the Leiden University Medical Center between 1995 and 2000 are included in our study. We completed a follow-up of 138 patients with squamous cell carcinoma of the lung and 77 patients with an adenocarcinoma of the lung. Patient and tumor characteristics are recorded from the medical records whereas information about venous thrombotic events is collected through the Anticoagulation Clinics. In order to accurately assess the histological diagnosis, tissue samples have been revised by an experienced pathologist.

Mean follow up of the patients with squamous cell carcinoma and adenocarcinoma was 1.46 years until the development of a VTE, death or the end of the study. In the group of patients with squamous cell cancer we found 9 cases (incidence: 41.9/1000/yr) of VTE whereas in the group of patients with adenocarcinoma 8 cases (incidence: 77.7/1000/yr) occurred. The age- and sex-adjusted hazard ratio was 1.4 (CI 95%: 0.7-4.4). These results suggest that the risk of a VTE is higher in patients with an adenocarcinoma than in patients with squamous cell carcinoma, although the difference is not striking.

PO 20
Bilateral Deep-Vein Thrombosis and Cancer: Prospective Study of 92 Patients

A BURA, B BIENVENU, N CAILLEUX, P LEGE, H BOCCALON, JN FIESSINGER, H LEVESQUE, J EMMERICH*
Service de Médecine Vasculaire, Hôpital Européen Georges Pompidou, Paris, Service de Médecine Interne, Rouen, Service de Médecine Vasculaire, Toulouse, France.

The association between bilateral deep-vein thrombosis (DVT) and cancer has been previously described in a single retrospective study. The aim of our study was to confirm this association in a prospective study of 92 patients consecutively followed in three departments of Vascular Medicine. The population consisted of 47 (51%) men and 45 (49%) women. Mean age was 68 years. Twentythree percent (23%) of patients had a previous history of DVT, and 41% had PE in association with the recent episode of venous thromboembolism. Twentythree patients (25% of the total) had a known active cancer at the time of acute DVT and unknown malignancy was detected in 16 patients (17%). For the patients without known cancer after hospital discharge the mean follow-up was 10.5 months; among them none had a cancer which appeared during this period. The total percentage of cancer associated with bilateral DVT was 42%. Overall cancer was more commonly found in patients with idiopathic DVT as compared with patients with known risk factors for DVT (25/46 vs 14/46). Total number of deaths was 19 (21%) after a mean follow-up of 8.4 months for the whole population. Our data confirm the results of our previous retrospective study. A particularly careful clinical examination for cancer should be performed when the diagnosis of bilateral DVT is objectively done. The usefulness of an extensive screening for the detection of occult malignancy has still to be demonstrated due to the poor prognosis of bilateral DVT observed in this study and to the fact that the majority of cancer in this situation are already known or easily found at the time of acute event.

PO 21
High Incidence of Thrombosis Using G-CSF in the Treatment of Chemotherapy-Induced Neutropenia

E CORTESI, A MANCUSO, L MOSCETTI, R SALTARELLI, M PALMA*
Cattedra di Oncologia Medica, Dipartimento di Medicina Sperimentale e Patologia, Università La Sapienza, Rome, Italy

Background: G-CSF is widely used as potent myelopoietic stimulators. However, its activity is not restricted to the myelopoietic system and several observations suggest that G-CSF could interfere with the hemostatic balance. The prevalence of thrombosis in cancer patients has been estimated as up to 15%. In order to assess the interaction between G-CSF and hemostasis, a retrospective analysis was performed on 409 patients treated with G-CSF and chemotherapy from 1996 to 2000. **Patients & Methods**: 287 patients were females and 122 were males, the mean age was 63.4 years, (range 43-76). No significant risk factors were detected. All patients had normal renal, hepatic and hematologic functions and were divided in three groups according to the number of total treatments with subcutaneous G-CSF at the standard dosage of 5 mg/kg. In the first cohort (A) (n=188, 46%) patients were treated with 1 to 5 administrations of G-CSF, while the second (B) (n=135, 33%) and third cohorts (C) (n=86, 21%) received from 6 to 10, and over 10 administrations, respectively. Thrombosis events occurred in 154 patients (37.65%) distributed as follows: Cohort (A):

18.18%, Cohort (B): 25.32%, Cohort (C): 54.49%. **Results**: Thromboembolic complications of central venous catheter were observed in 57.8% of patients, while thrombosis of intra-arterial catheter and deep vein thrombosis were respectively 3.25% and 31.8% of cases. Seven patients (4.55%) developed subclavian vein thrombosis, pulmonary embolization in 1.95% of cases, and in only one patient (0.65%) autopsy revealed acute multifocal cerebral venous thrombosis. **Conclusions**: These observations indicate that G-CSF administration may induce a higher risk of thrombosis, and a careful monitoring of the venous circolation should be done.

PO 22
Acquired and Genetic Thrombotic Risk Factor in a Young Woman with Recurrent TVP: A Case Report

P DI MICCO, A. NIGLIO, MR DIADEMA, F DE VITA, M D'UVA*
V° Division General Medicine, Second University of Naples, Italy

M.R., a 37 years old woman, was admitted to our Division with a proxymal deep venous thrombosis of left leg. Thrombosis was confirmed by clinical examination, ecocolordoppler examination, d-dimer plasma levels (5.7 ng/dl) and F1+2 plasma concentration (3.9 nM). Anamnesis visualized two previous TVP. Physical examination showed a small mammalian swelling and a following biopsy revealed a breast cancer. Oncological staging didn't show lymph nodes involvement or metastasis: a surgical treatment was performed. Yet, laboratory tests to search familiar haemostasis abnormalities showed also a protein S deficit (total protein S antigen: 38%). These data show not only the relevance of high thrombotic risk in people carrying genetic haemostasis abnormalities, but also the relevance of acquired cause of thrombosis as cancer: cancer, in fact, is recognized as the most common acquired cause of thrombosis also in non advanced stage. Moreover, our case shows the contemporaneousness of genetic and acquired thrombotic risk factor in people affected by recurrent deep venous thrombosis.

PO 23
The Differences between Clinical and Autopsy Outcomes in Thrombosis and Bleeding in Malignancies

M PENKA, I PENKA*
Masaryk University Hospital, Brno - Bohunice, Czech Republic

Coagulation disorders allow to divide the tumours into three categories: 1) with thrombin generation, 2) with expression of urokinase type of plasminogen activator and 3) with both or none of the above mentioned mechanisms. As clinical symptomatology of coagulopathies thrombosis, bleeding or thrombosis and bleeding - thrombohemorhagic syndrome can be observed. The blood coagulation investigation includes global tests - PT, APTT, TT, level of fibrinogen and plasmatic factors and inhibitors. Specific examination represents the detection of hypercoagulation markers: fibrin monomers, fibrinopeptide A, F1+2, thrombin-antithrombin complexes. Fibrinolytic activity is evaluated by D-dimer and fibrinogen-fibrin degradation products assays and by the time of euglobulin fibrinolysis test. The type of the tumour and results of laboratory tests are the starting point for the prophylaxis and the treatment. The useful treatment of coagulation disorders decreases not only thrombotic and haemorrhagic complications but also improves the global results of the complex care in oncology. We analysed 118 malignant patients, who died on malignancy in our hospital. They all underwent the autopsy. We estimated the incidence of thrombotic and haemorrhagic events, their laboratory diagnostics and compared clinical as well as autopsy findings. We focused our attention on the differences between the clinical diagnosis and autopsy outcomes. The incidence of clinical symptomatology of blood coagulation disorders corresponded to literature data. The differences between clinical and autopsy outcomes were found in hemorragic group in 42% and in thrombotic group in 58% of patients. The cause of death were bleeding and thrombosis in 7% of all the patients. Conclusion:the discrepancy of clinical and autopsy findings requests more sophisticated diagnostic attitudes and more scheduled approach such as protocolar prophylactic and treatment regimes for an improvement of the results of the global care in oncology.

PO 24
Mechanisms for Acquired Activated Protein C Resistance in Cancer Patients

G SARIG[1], Y MICHAELI[2,3], N LANIR[1], B BRENNER[1,3], N HAIM[2,3]*
[1]Thrombosis and Hemostasis Unit and [2]Department of Oncology, Rambam Medical Center and the [3]Bruce Rappaport Faculty of Medicine, Technion-Israel Institute of Technology, Haifa, Israel

Acquired activated protein C resistance (APCR) is common in cancer patients and may increase the risk of venous thromboembolism in these patients. In order to study the mechanisms for acquired APCR in cancer patients, we prospectively evaluated coagulation factors II, V, VIII and protein S levels, as well as presence of antiphospholipid antibodies, in patients with solid tumors without thrombosis. APCR (APC-sensitivity ratio<2.0) without factor V Leiden was documented in 9/70 (13%) of cancer patients compared to none of controls (P=0.03). APCR was not associated with low levels of free protein S (3% in patients vs. 4% in controls, P=0.7) nor with presence of antiphospholipid antibodies (5% in patients vs 6% in controls, P=0.65). In addition, there was no difference in prothrombin levels between patients and controls (99 ± 13 u/dl vs 96 ± 16 u/dl). Elevated levels (>150 u/dl) of coagulation factors V and VIII were significantly more common in cancer patients compared to controls (21% vs. 3% and 40% vs. 0%, P=0.03 and P=0.02, respectively). APC sensitivity ratios in cancer patients inversely correlated with factor V and factor VIII levels, but did not correlate with factor II nor with protein S levels. Our preliminary results suggest that in cancer patients APCR without factor V Leiden may result from elevated levels of coagulation factors V and VIII. The potential implications of these findings on thrombotic risk in cancer patients require further investigation.

PO 25
The Prevalence of Inherited Thrombophilia in Patients with Cancer: Preliminary Findings

S BATTISTELLI[1], M RANALLI[1], S BATTISTINI[2], T AMATO[2], F ROVIELLO[2], L SABATINI[3], D MARRELLI[4], S MANCINI[1]*
[1]Istituto di Chirurgia Generale e Specialità Chirurgiche, [2]Istituto di Scienze Neurologiche, [3]U.O. di Ematologia e Coagulazione, [4]Istituto di Scienze Chirurgiche; Policlinico LE SCOTTE, Università di Siena, Italy

Purpose: Cancer patients are at increased risk of venous thromboembolism. The pathogenetic mechanisms for the production of the hypercoagulable state in cancer are not entirely understood but surely "acquired thrombophilia" plays an important role. Little is known about the association of "inherited thrombophilia" and cancer hypercoagulability. The aim of this study was to examine in cancer patients the frequency of the most common inherited coagulation defects associated with venous thromboembolism, such as antithrombin III, protein S and protein C deficiency, factor V Leiden mutation (G1691A), prothrombin G20210A variant and 5-10 methylenetetrahydrofolate reductase (MTHFR) C677T polimorphysm. **Subjects and Methods**: Fifty consecutive cancer patients (mean age 68 years) with gastrointestinal or pelvic primary solid neoplasm and 50 healthy controls matched for age, were enrolled in the study. Antithrombin III and protein C activity were measured by automated chromogenic method, protein S activity by the clotting method. Factor V Leiden mutation and MTHFR C677T polimorphysm were determined by polymerase chain reaction (PCR) and restriction analysis, prothrombin G20210A variant was evaluated by Allele-Specific PCR. **Results**: In cancer group the frequency of inherited coagulation defects was the following: protein S deficiency 6%, protein C deficiency 2%; individuals carrying allele A of Factor V Leiden 2% (GA genotype), allele A of prothrombin G20210A variant 10% (GA genotype) and allele T of MTHFR C677T polimorphysm 74% (44% CT and 30% TT genotype). No cases of antithrombin III deficiency were observed. In control group the frequency of inherited coagulation defects were the following: protein S deficiency 2%; individuals carrying allele A of Factor V Leiden 2% (GA genotype), allele A of prothrombin G20210A variant

4% (GA genotype) and allele T of MTHFR C677T polimorphysm 74% (48% CT and 26% TT genotype). No cases of antithrombin III and protein C deficiency were observed. The frequency of various risk factors was not significantly different between the two groups. **Conclusion**: In cancer patients with solid tumors the prevalence of inherited thrombophilia seems not differ from that of control subjects. Further studies on a greater sample size are undergoing to confirm these preliminary findings and to understand their clinical significance.

PO 26
Activated Protein C Resistance in Nonmetastatic Gastric Cancer Patients

P DI MICCO, A NIGLIO, G CHIRICO, D DI GIUSEPPE, F RUSSO, A FEDERICO, M ROMANO, R TORELLA*
V° Division General Medicine, Second University of Naples, Italy

Introduction Cancer is the most common acquired cause of thrombosis, and thromboembolic complications are frequent in cancer patients. Moreover, thromboembolic complications represent the second cause of death in malignancy. Furthermore gastrointestinal malignancies are associated with hypercoagulable state in advanced stage and this seems to be related also to an acquired protein C resistance (APCr). The aim of the study is to investigate APCr in nonmetastatic gastric cancer patients. **Patients & methods** We selected 11 patients affected by gastric cancer (9 males and 2 females, mean age 48 +/- 8 years, 10 intestinal type and 1 diffuse type) and studied their hypercoagulable state and 20 healthy subjects as control group. We measured in both group PT, aPTT, fibrinogen, APCr (according to the method described by Bertina) and F1+2 as marker of thrombin generation. **Results** No differences were assessed in PT and aPTT values. Fibrinogen plasma concentration was higher in cancer patients than in controls (532 +/- 31 mg/dl vs 295 +/- 34 mg/dl, p<0.01) as F1+2 (4.12 +/-0.82 nM vs 0.77 +/- 0.12 nM, p<0.01. Finally no differences were recognized in APCr in both group (0.96 +/- 0.11 vs 0.95 +/- 0.13). **Discussion** Hypercoagulable state is common in gastrointestinal cancer patients and an acquired APCr could explain it in advanced stage as reported in the Literature. Yet, in nonmetastatic gastric cancer our data showed that hypercoagulable state present in natural history of the disease not seems to be related to APCr.

PO 27
Activation of Coagulation in Cancer: A Mathematical Model

*AA SBIGNEV, MA KHANIN**
Moscow, Russia

The purpose of this research was to develop a mathematical model of coagulation system dynamic and steady state in cancer, and to study coagulation initiation. Model involves following physiological processes. Tumor cells express tissue factor (TF), cancer procoagulants and release cytokines: interleukin-1beta, tissue necrosis factor (TNF-alpha) and vascular endothelial growth factor (VEGF), that is important in coagulation initiation. Then endothelial cells express TF, while thrombomodulin (TM) expression by endothelial cells simultaneously decreases. As a result, coagulation process is triggered and fibrin is generated. Besides, coagulation (factors VII, V, VIII, IX, X, XI, II, I, PC activation and tenase, prothrombinase, TF-VII and TF-thrombin complexes formation, inhibitory effect-antithrombin III, PCa, TFPI-tissue factor inhibitor, CI inhibitor) and fibrinolytic (plasminogen activation by t-PA-tissue plasminogen activator and u-PA-urokinase plasminogen activator, and its inhibition by PAI-1 and PAI-2) processes are involved into the mathematical model. Thus, we considered enzymatic cascade, positive and negative feedbacks and complexes formation (second order biochemical reactions). Mathematical model is presented by a set of coupled, nonlinear, first order ordinary differential equations (balance equation for all factors, which participated in processes). In this model, Michaelis-Menten kinetics was used. Solution of the set of equations was obtained by numerical Runge-Kutta method. Mathematical modeling of coagulation and fibrinolysis dynamics permitted us to establish the threshold effect in coagulation activation in cancer. Thus, thrombosis can be realized only for sufficiently large tumors.

PO 28
Von Willebrand Factor (VWF) in Autologous Stem Cell Transplantation

*A LATTUADA, A ROSTI, E SACCHI, C CALZAROSSA, U RUSSO, E ROSSI**
Ospedale Sacco, Milan, Italy

Hemopoietic cells reside predominantly in the bone marrow and can be mobilized in large numbers in blood by the administration of CSF (Colony Stimulating Factor). Apheresis products containing CSF-mobilized peripheral-blood cells are now widely used instead of bone marrow for autologous transplantation, because the hematopoietic recovery is faster with the use of peripheral-blood cells than with the use of bone marrow. This procedure requires high-dose chemotherapy with consequent marrow displasia and endothelial damage by mechanisms not yet well clarified. Thrombotic events are frequent in these patients, Venous-Occlusive Disease (VOD), Thrombotic Thrombocitopenic Purpura (TTP) being the most important complications. In TTP, platelet adhesion to the damaged subendothelium could justify the prolonged thrombocytopenia, vWF being the most important protein involved in platelet adhesion and aggregation. With this background, we studied 6 patients during autologous stem cell transplantation to evaluate the change of concentration and activity of vWF, the vWF cleaving protease and platelet count. The results (mean ± SD) observed before (B) and after (A) high dose chemioterapy (HDC) and before and after reinfusion (R) are:

	vWF:Ag %	vWF-protease %	vWF:CB %	Plts $10^3/\mu l$
B HDC	97 ± 33	107 ± 22	64 ± 22	333 ± 97
A HDC	112 ± 36	92 ± 20	98 ± 10	220 ± 33
B R	159 ± 37	76 ± 24	186 ± 19	177 ± 85
A R	156 ± 25	75 ± 22	197 ± 47	46 ± 18

Conclusions: in autologous stem cell transplantation the increased concentration and activity of vWF could explain the occurence of TTP and VOD, and justify the prolonged thrombocytopenia and platelet transfusion refractoriness.

PO 29
Predictive Model for the Development of Veno-Occlusive Disease (VOD) Following Stem Cell Transplantation (SCT)

T ZUCKERMAN, I GAVISH, I AVIVI, A ERAN, I BEN-YEHUDA, E SABO, N LANIR, JM ROWE, B BRENNER*
Department of Hematology & Bone Marrow Transplantation, Rambam Medical Center, Pathology Institute, Carmel Hospital, Haifa, Israel

There are substantial controversies regarding frequency, pathogenesis, and risk factors and treatment of VOD following SCT. The aim of this study was to prospectively examine clinical and laboratory predictive parameters of VOD in a large transplant referral center. Study design: 161 consecutive patients admitted for SCT between 12/1998 and 5/2000 including 117 patients with autologous and 44 with allogeneic transplants. VOD prophylaxis consisted of ursodil for the autologous group and ursodil with heparin for the allogeneic group. Patients who developed severe VOD were treated with defibrotide 10-40 mg/kg/day for at least 14 days. Blood was drawn weekly before and after SCT. Samples were analyzed for von-Willebrand factor (vWF), soluble thrombomodulin (TM), factor V Leiden (FVL), factor II G20210A (PTM), and MTHFR 677TT. **Results**: 24 patients (14.9%) developed VOD, 21 according to Baltimore criteria, 3 according to Seattle criteria. 65% had mild to moderate VOD and 35% severe *VOD, with 47% mortality in the severe group. Of the allogeneic SCT, 48% developed VOD as compared to only 2.5% in the autologous SCT (OR 13.4; p=0.00001). TM levels were higher on day +7 (p=0.03) and +14 (p=0.003) in the VOD group, while vWF levels did not differ between the VOD and non-VOD groups. FVL, PTM and MTHFR 677TT mutations were not associated with development of VOD. By univariate analysis: allogeneic BMT, treatment with busulfan and TM levels on days +7, +14 were significantly associated with VOD (p=0.00001, p=0.0005, p=0.03, p=0.003, respectively). By multivariate analysis, the independent significant predictors of VOD were allogeneic SCT, higher CD34 kg/body weight, diagnosis of AML/ALL and TM level on day +7 (p=0.0002, p=0.02, p=0.03, p=0.0001, respectively), resulting in sensitivity of 85% and specificity of 74%. **Conclusion**: This combined clinical and laboratory model may serve as a predictive tool for development of VOD following SCT. Thrombophilic polymorphism is not a contributing factor for the development of VOD.

PO 30
Changes of Coagulable Hemostatic Mechanism During Cytostatic Treatment of Patients with Breast Cancer

D PETROVIÆ, D JOVANOVIÆ*
Institutski put br.4, Sremska Kamenica, Yugoslavia

During the course of cytostatic treatment of the patients with breast cancer an increased incidence of thromboembolic complications was recognized. We examined the effect of CMF protocol cytostatic therapy to hemostatic parameters in patients with localized and disseminated breast cancer. The study included 30 patients with stage II and 30 patients with stage IV of breast cancer. At the beginning and at the end of the first sequence of cytostatic treatment of CMF protocol the following hemostatic parameters were determined: number of thrombocytes, fibrinogen level, protein C and ATIII activity, TAT level, D-dimer, PT, APTT, TT and euglobulin time. After CMF therapy, patients with stage II of breast cancer manifested a significant decrease in the number of thrombocytes ($p<0.01$), PC and ATIII activity ($p<0.01$) and an increase in TAT level ($p<0.01$). In patients with disseminated breast cancer CMF therapy resulted in an increased level of changes in hemostatic parameters (decrease in the number of thrombocytes, decrease in PC and ATIII activity with an increased level of TAT and D-dimer, and reducing of PT, APTT and TT). Our results suggest that the application of cytostatic therapy incites hypecoagulable condition in breast cancer patients. Pathophysiological mechanism of hypercoagulable condition incited after CMF therapy has still to be cleared up.

PO 31
Bleeding and Thrombosis in Acute Promyelocytic Leukemia - A Single Center Experience in 29 Patients

N DALLY, R HOFFMAN, G SARIG, N LANIR, JM ROWE, B BRENNER*
Department of Hematolgoy and Bone Marrow Transplantation, Rambam Medical Center, Haifa, Israel

Thrombosis and hemorrhage are common features in acute promyelocytic leukemia (APL). However, because APL is relatively uncommon, most reported series represent multicenter studies. We report the hemorrhagic and thrombotic events at presentation and during induction in 29 consecutive APL patients treated in a single referral center from 1994 to 2001. Threatening bleeding manifestations occurred in 9 (31%) patients; 8 (27%) had diffuse alveolar hemorrhage (one patient died), 2 had cerebral hemorrhage, one had intra abdominal hemorrhage and two women suffered severe vaginal bleeding. Four patients (13%) had severe thrombotic events. Two cerebral sagittal sinus thrombosis, one pulmonary embolism and one had subclavian vein thrombosis. Two other patients had pseudo-tumor cerebri. Three of 6 patients with thrombotic events were found to have thrombophilia. Two patients suffered from combined severe bleeding and thrombosis. The most consistent hemostatic abnormality was decreased (<150mg/dl) fibrinogen level, found in 17 (58%), PTT was normal in all patients. A mildly prolonged PT was observed in 11/29 (38%). Mean platelet count was $43x10^9/L$ (range $5-151x10^9/L$). Bleeding complications did not correlate with hemostatic parameters. Despite treatment with ATRA and intensive supportive care, hemorrhagic and thrombotic events remain a major problem at presentation and during induction of APL patients. While hemostatic parameters do not predict hemorrhage, thrombosis is often associated with thrombophilia.

PO 32
Thrombotic Thrombocytopenic Purpura (TTP) in Cancer Patients Receiving Chemotherapy: Evidence of Increased Nitric Oxide Production

C PORTA [1]*, E BOBBIO-PALLAVICINI [2], F PIOVELLA [1,3], A NATALIZI [1,3], S FERRARI [1], L LIBRE [3], M DANOVA [1]
[1]Medicina Interna ed Oncologia Medica, [3]Servizio Malattie Tromboemboliche, Università degli Studi di Pavia, IRCCS Policlinico San Matteo, Pavia, and [2]Oncologia Medica ed Ematologia, Ospedale Maggiore di Crema, Italy

Although rare, the occurrence of TTP in cancer patients receiving chemotherapy has been well established. We report on three new cases of TTP developing in cancer patients receiving different chemotherapy drugs. Moreover, using a sensitive HPLC method, we evaluated the stable nitric oxide (NO) end-products nitrite (NO_2) and nitrate (NO_3) in the plasma of these patients. For HPLC analysis, a Supelcosil LC-18 column and a Supelguard LC-18 precolumn were used. HPLC conditions were chosen as follows: eluent, n-octylamine 0.01 mol/L; flow rate, 1.2 mL/min; detection UV 205 nm; retention times for NO_2 and NO_3 amounted to 9.3 min and to 15.1 min, respectively; finally, the detection limits were 2 mmol/L NO_2 and 7 mmol/L NO_3. As expected, no detectable levels of NO_2 were shown in the plasma of the three patients. Indeed, only NO_3 represents the final metabolite of NO in the blood. Thus, NO_3 titers in the three chemotherapy-related TTP cases were 184.3, 218.28 and 185.0 mmol/L, respectively. These figures were fairly higher than those previously observed in 29 idiopathic TTP patients (average: 25.86 mmol/L) and in 29 sex- and age-matched healthy controls (average: 24.23 mmol/L). This suggests a severe endothelial dysfunction in our oncologic patients who developed TTP. The observed increased release of NO_3 could be interpreted as the consequence of massive disruption of endothelial integrity, with consequent passive NO release in vivo, or as an active compensatory mechanism the endothelium tries to compensate for diffuse microvascular occlusion. The two mechanisms may also be associated, but the normal titers of NO end-products in de novo TTP suggest that the former mechanism may be the more important one, at least in cancer chemotherapy-related TTP.

PO 33
Effectiveness of Low Molecular Weight Heparin (LMWH) in Cancer-Related Disseminated Intravascular Coagulation (DIC). A Case Report

F VITALE*, D PRIOLO, D SAMBATARO, P COLINA, F FERRAU'
Division of Medical Oncology, Ospedale S.Vincenzo, Taormina, Italy

Introduction: Acute DIC is one of the most critical complications induced by cancer-related factors or the same antineoplastic treatment. The use of LMWH is well defined for the treatment of thromboembolic disease and thrombosis prophylaxis in cancer patients, while much remains to be understood about their safety and effectiveness in the therapy of DIC. **Case report**: A 60-year old female patient affected by an adenocarcinoma of the right lung metastatic to contralateral lung and bone, previously treated with two lines of chemotherapy, was admitted to our Department with severe emesis, consciousness deficit and arterial hypertension; the last chemotherapy cycle had been administered more then three months before. Magnetic resonance showed bilateral cerebral metastases and hydrocephalus; therapy with dexamethasone and i.v. mannitol did not obtain significant clinical benefit. Few days later, macroscopic haematuria occurred; laboratory findings witnessed the presence of an acute DIC (platelets count: 34,000/microliter, fibrinogenemia: 79 mg/dL; prothrombin time: 30 sec.; D-Dimer elevation: 550 mcg/L). The patient was treated with subcutaneously nadroparin calcium (92.7 U/kg twice daily) and a single supply of fresh frozen plasma. After 24 hours, fibrinogenemia and prothrombin time were normalized, platelets count began to increase, and then the bleeding stopped. A week later platelets count was 110,000/microliter, without further fresh plasma or platelets transfusion. Ten days later the patient died because of worsening of hydrocephalus. **Discussion**: The occurrence of acute DIC is a dramatic as well as common feature in cancer patients with advanced disease and the treatment requires considerable resource implications for the oncologists. The optimal management is controversial. Among the different treatment, the classical unfractionated heparin (UFH) continuous infusion is controversial, mainly for the risk of worsening of hemorragic syndrome. Various studies have stressed that LMWH therapy is handy, safer and more cost-effective than intravenous UFH for the cancer-related hypercoagulability complications (predictably high absorption rate, prolonged duration of action when given subcutaneously, no needing of continuous intravenous infusion and laboratory monitoring). Our report suggests that LMWH use can improve the severe DIC state induced by disseminated solid tumors. Further thorough investigations are required to explore the potential of LMWH for acute DIC treatment and/or prophylaxis.

PO 34
Cancer-Related Mild Disseminated Intravascular Coagulation (Mild DIC): A Possible Role for Nadroparin Therapy

F VITALE[1], D PRIOLO[1], S ROTONDO[2], M MATTINA[1], F FERRAU'[1]*
[1]Division of Medical Oncology, [2]Division of Internal Medicine, Ospedale S.Vincenzo, Taormina, Italy

Background Mild DIC frequently occurs in advanced malignancies, but the diagnosis is often difficult because of lack of consensus about the appropriate clinical and laboratory criteria of diagnosis. Laboratory findings include borderline or slow progressive dropping of platelets count (pc), D-dimer elevation, normal or moderately deranged level of prothrombin time (PT), activated partial thromboplastin time (aPTT), fibrinogen and antithrombin III. Bleeding is not common but mild DIC can progress to overt acute DIC. No clear therapeutical guidelines are defined. **Patients & Methods** Between May 2000 and June 2001 we have tested the effectiveness of nadroparin calcium in nine cancer patients with mild DIC (5 males; median age 65 years, range 52-81), affected by advanced lung (3), pancreas (3), breast (1), prostate (1) and ovary (1) carcinoma. The elegibility criteria included: metastatic cancer not pretreated with chemotherapy or last course administered at least eight weeks before thrombocytopenia diagnosis; D-dimer elevation; pc drop observed for at least five days and not more than 12,000/microliter/die; fibrinogenemia and antithrombin III level within or slightly under the normal level; PT and aPTT unchanged or mildly prolonged; red blood cells fragmentation tested in the blood samples; normal leucocyte count; pc rising within 36 hours after the time of heparinization. A first group of five patients had an initial pc more than 100,000/microliter; a second group of four patients had an initial pc less than 100,000/microliter. Nadroparin was administered subcutaneously, at dose 100 U.I./Kg once daily. **Results** In the first group of patients, platelet count progressively returned to normal, after a median of 5 days; with regard to second group, platelet count increased over 100,000/microliter but full normalization was not obtained. All the nine patients remained free from further exhacerbation of DIC at least for the following six weeks after nadroparin therapy starting. No relevant side effect related to nadroparin was recorded. **Conclusions** Nadroparin calcium seems able to inhibit the decrease in platelet count and to improve the mild DIC state in progressive solid tumors, thus preventing or at least delaying the onset of overt DIC in these patients

PO 35
Hypercoagulability Due to Phenotypic APC Resistance in Primitive Cerebral Lymphoma

D DE LUCIA[1], F DE FRANCESCO[1], R MAROTTA[1], G MAISTO[1], M SORRENTINO[1], ML PAPA[2]*
[1]Institute of General Pathology and Oncology; II University of Naples, [2]Laboratory of Haemostasis and Thrombosis; San Giovanni Bosco Hospital, Naples, Italy

Primary central nervous system non-Hodgkin's lymphoma represents a rare pathology. Thrombosis is the most frequent complication and the second cause of death in patients with malignant disease. Recently, a new mechanism of hereditary thrombophilia characterized by a poor response to activated protein C (APC-resistance) has been identified. Resistance to APC is usually linked to a factor V (FV) gene mutation changing an Arg 506 to a Gln in the APC cleavage site. In our study, we aimed at investigating the presence of

APC-resistance and other markers of hypercoagulability in 15 selected patients with a diagnosis of primitive cerebral lymphoma who had suffered from an ischemic episode of TIA and/or stroke. Twenty-two healthy subjects acted as a control group. We measured APC resistance, natural clotting inhibitors, (F1+2) and FPA according to international guidelines. Genomic DNA was extracted from peripheral white blood cells and a PCR was performed to amplify genomic exon 10/intron 10 region of FV gene to search for Arg506 to Gln point mutation. Our results showed that 9 out of 15 patients had a poor response to APC (<0.70, which represents the cut-off point in our general population) without deficiencies in natural clotting inhibitors. All patients had high plasma levels of F1+2 and FPA compared to those found in healthy subjects (2.65±0.75 nM vs. 0.40±0.35 nM; 3.95±0.85 nmol/L vs 1.6±0.8 nmol/L, respectively). In 7 patients resistance to APC was not associated to a FV gene defect demonstrating that such phenomenon may occur also as an acquired condition. However, the patients with resistance to APC showed the highest plasma values in F1+2 and FPA. In cerebral lymphoma with hypercoagulability the resistance to APC is not caused by the FV Arg506->Gln mutation (77%). APC resistance not caused by this FV gene defect may be a risk factor for thrombophilia in this selected population.

PO 36
A Morphological and Functional Analysis of Platelet VEGF in Cancer Patients

R SALGADO [1,2], I BENOY [1,2], J BOGERS [2], R WEYTJENS [1], P VERMEULEN [1,2], M HOYLAERTS [3], L DIRIX [1], E VAN MARCK [2]*

[1]Angiogenesis Group, Oncological Centre, St-Augustinus Hospital, [2]Department of Pathology, University of Antwerp, Wilrijk, [3]Center for Molecular and Vascular Biology, University of Leuven, Belgium

The growth of primary tumours is dependent on angiogenesis. The switch to the angiogenic phenotype involves changes in the local equilibrium of cytokines with either pro- or anti-angiogenic properties. Vascular Endothelial Growth Factor (VEGF) is one of the major positive regulators of tumour angiogenesis. Recent evidence suggests that platelets are the main contributors of serum VEGF. In this study we analysed ultrastructurally and with immunofluorescence techniques, the topographical localisation of VEGF in platelets. An alpha-granule and membranous VEGF-localisation was identified. In 34 untreated metastatic breast cancer patients, 21 patients with locoregional breast cancer and 24 healthy individuals, we analysed serum VEGF (SVEGF) and plasma VEGF (PVEGF) levels. The mean circulating SVEGF levels for the healthy controls, localised breast cancer group and patients with metastasis were 97.2 pg/ml (med.: 77 pg/ml; SD= 71.23), 330.5 pg/ml (med.: 279.3; SD= 249.1) and 405.5 pg/ml (med.: 331.8; SD= 249.1) respectively (P<0.0001; Kruskal-Wallis test). Correlation analysis between SVEGF and platelets reached borderline significance in both the untreated (r= 0.42, P= 0.07) as well as in the metastatic breast cancer group (r= 0.32; P= 0.07). The calculated SVEGF load per platelet rose from 0.39 pg/10^6 platelets in the control population, 1.22 pg/10^6 platelets till 1.79 pg/10^6 for platelets in patients with metastasis (P<0.0001; Kruskal-Wallis test). Mean PVEGF levels were 13.7 pg/ml (med.: 12.55 pg/ml; SD= 9.2) for the control group, 32.12 pg/ml (med.: 30.25 pg/ml; SD=16.25) for the localised breast cancer group and 54.78 pg/ml (med.: 43.75 pg/ml; SD= 35.98) for the metastasis group (P<0.0001; Kruskal-Wallis test). The correlation coefficients between PVEGF and the VEGF load/platelet were 0.57 (P=0.004), 0.60 (P=0.005) and 0.57 (P=0.0001) for the healthy control population, for the localised and advanced breast cancer group. In 12 patients with colon cancer we analysed with immunohistochemistry for the platelet membrane glycocalicin platelet adherence and aggregation on tumoural endothelium. Our results suggest that platelets are important in the storage of circulating VEGF. The progressive accumulation of VEGF in platelets according to tumoural progression may be due to endocytosis of tumour cell produced-VEGF and/or enhancement of VEGF synthesis in platelet precursors, the megakaryocytes. Platelets may subsequently adhere on tumoural endothelium and release, concomitantly with aggregation, the higher VEGF load and thereby provide an additional stimulus for ongoing intra-tumoural angiogenesis.

PO 37
PAI-5G/5G Allele Distribution in Neoplastic Patients with Colon Cancer

M CIGOLINI [1]*, S ZEMINIAN[1], D BARANA [2], C OLIANI [2], C CARDINALE [3], PF PIGNATTI [3]
[1]Internal Medicine, Arzignano Hospital, Arzignano, [2]Experimental Medicine Dept, and [3]Maternal/Pediatric Dept, University of Verona, Verona, Italy

Type-1 Plasminogen Activator Inhibitor (PAI-1) is the major circulating inhibitor of fibrinolysis. Since many years, PAI-1 is known to play an important role in different cellular pathways. Several studies suggest that PAI-1 activity influences neoplasm progression and metastasis capacity. Degradation and remodelling of normal tissue and tumor tissue is controlled by limited proteolysis of extracellular matrix. Circulating plasma PAI-1 levels have been related to a common single base pair guanosine insertion/deletion polymorphism (4G/5G) which has been shown to be an enhancer/repressor binding site in the promoter region of the PAI-1 gene, that also influences PAI-1 plasma activity. Our interest has been to analyse the polymorphism distribution of the PAI-1 promoter and its association with neoplastic patients with new diagnosis of colon cancer (n=86) without family history positive for cardiovascular disease. As control population, we choosed 107 unknown random healthy subjects. Genomic DNA was extracted from 10 mL of whole peripheral blood following standards methods. PAI-1 4G/5G polymorphism was detected after PCR by restriction digestion of product. In reason of the hypotesized role for PAI-1 in fybrinolitic activity regulation and in extracellular matrix degradation during tumor invasion and metastatic diffusion, we compared genotype distribution between patients with colon neoplasm and control population without colon cancer, and we observed that there was a statistically significant difference between the two groups (allele 5G/5G neoplastic 10.5% vs non neoplastic 29.9%, p=0.0045). In our opinion, knowing if our colon cancer patient is homozygous 5G/5G could help planning our therapeutical strategy more aggressively in attempt to stop metastatic diffusion. In conclusion, we conclude that plasminogen activator inhibitor type 1 (PAI-1) 5G/5G genotype is more frequent in colon cancer patients than in controls.

PO 38
Lipase, Basic Fibroblast Growth Factor, Heparanase and Cancer: Linking an Altered Biochemical Profile with Thrombosis, Angiogenesis and Metastasis

C PORTA [1]*, G DIANI [2], M DANOVA [1], M BARONE [3], S SERAFINI [3], F PIOVELLA [3]
[1]Medicina Interna ed Oncologia Medica, [2]Servizio di Analisi Biochimico-Cliniche, [3]Servizio Malattie Tromboemboliche, IRCCS Policlinico San Matteo, Pavia, Italy

Recent reports suggested that the biochemical profile characterized by increased lipase and normal amylase titers might be an early finding of a metastasizing malignant neoplasm. We have assayed both lipase and amylase in the sera of 500 consecutive cancer patients with no clinical or instrumental signs of neoplastic pancreatic involvement. Serum lipase activity was assayed using a commercial kit. Ninety-three patients - i.e., 18.3% - were thus identified. Despite its relevant limitations, this retrospective survey suggests that the presence of hyperlipasemia with normal amylasemia is a much more common event in cancer patients than it could be expected. Since heparanase, in addition to being involved in the remodelling of extracellular matrix and in the egress of cells from vasculature, may also regulate angiogenesis, tissue repair and lipid metabolism by releasing heparan sulfate-bound growth factors and enzymes such as basic fibroblast growth factor (bFGF) and lipoprotein lipase, we wondered on the possible involvement of heparanases in the biological phenomenon we observed. Indeed, if heparanase-induced degradation of extracellular matrix, with concurrent release of pro-metastatic and pro-angiogenetic growth factors, is an early event in the process of tumor invasion and metastasis, then release of heparan sulfate-bound lipase could be the cause of the elevation in serum lipase associated with the development of distant metastases we have observed. To test this hypothesis, we titered bFGF on sera of the above 93 patients presenting with hyperlipasemia, finding elevated titers of this pro-angiogenetic cytokine. Indeed, bFGF titers in these patients were significantly higher than those observed in age- and sex-matched healthy controls; furthermore, bFGF and lipase titers were significantly correlated when analyzed by regression analysis. Even though preliminary, these results prompted us to actively pursue this field of investigation.

PO 39
The Role of Fibrinolysis in Chemotherapy Induced Hypercoagulability

CC KIRWAN, IJ AHMED, F TORELLA, CN MCCOLLUM, GJ BYRNE*
South Manchester University Hospital, Manchester, England.

Introduction: Venous thromboembolism (VTE) is common in cancer. During chemotherapy, VTE occurs in up to 17% of patients with advanced breast cancer. Chemotherapy induced hypercoagulability may occur through a reduction in fibrinolysis. Here we study the fibrinolytic molecules tissue-type plasminogen activator (tPA) and urokinase-type plasminogen activator (uPA). **Methods**: Serum tPA and uPA were measured before (baseline) and 1, 4, and 8 days, and 3 months after chemotherapy in 17 patients with advanced, and 17 patients with early, breast or colorectal carcinoma, receiving adjuvant therapy. **Results**: At baseline tPA was elevated in the advanced cancer group at 1634 (SD 865) pg/ml as compared to 1128 (SD 614) pg/ml in early cancer (p=0.053). There was no difference in uPA between the two groups: 0.67 (SD 0.38) ng/ml and 0.67 (SD 0.12) ng/ml respectively. In advanced cancer, mean tPA fell during the first week of chemotherapy, to a maximal 522 (SE 114) pg/ml below baseline at day 4, and rising to 183 (SE 249) pg/ml by 3 months. In early cancer, mean tPA increased in the week following chemotherapy to a maximum on day one of 282 (SE 158) pg/ml, but falling to 67(SE 118) pg/ml below baseline by 3 months. Mean uPA in advanced cancer demonstrated a minimal increase following chemotherapy, reaching a maximum of 0.063 (SE 0.032) ng/ml above baseline at day 4. By 3 months this had increased to 0.27 (SE 0.17) ng/ml. In early cancer, mean uPA on day 1 initially increased to 0.12 (SE 4.9) ng/ml: this returned to baseline by 3 months. However, these trends were not statistically significant.

PO 40
Pregnancy and Abortion in Women with Essential Thrombocythemia

A CANDONI[1], T MICHELUTTI[1], D DAMIANI[1], A SPEROTTO[1], A MICHELUTTI[1], M CERNO[1], R FANIN[1], M BACCARANI[2]*
[1]Division of Hematology, University Hospital, Udine, [2]Institute of Hematology and Medical Oncology "Seragnoli", University of Bologna, Italy

Essential Thrombocythemia (ET) is a chronic myeloproliferative disease (CMD) associated with an increased risk of thrombotic and haemorrhagic complications. Although ET usually occurs in an older age group, this disease may be observed in young adults and in these patients frequently it is detected incidentally. We report our experience in a specific group of young patients with ET: women in pregnancy. Between 1989 and 2000, 50 women younger than 45 years with ET were seen at our Department. Diagnosis was made according with the criteria of Polycythemia Vera Study Group. Among 50 women, 17 pregnancies occured in 12 patients. The median age at diagnosis of ET was 27 years (range 17-39) and 28 years (range 19-40) at the beginning of pregnancy; in 7/12 patients the disease was discovered incidentally and only 5/12 women were symptomatic. Platelet counts at diagnosis ranged from 650 to 1,750x10^9/L (median 800x10^9/L). Of the 17 pregnancies 7 (41%) resulted in live birth and 10 (59%) ended in spontaneous abortion (8/10 in the first trimester); all seven deliveries were uncomplicated. Only three patients had episodes of mild vaginal bleeding; no preeclampsia, preterm delivery and other complications, during postpartum period, were reported. Preconception platelet counts of pregnancies carried to term (median 850x10^9/L; range 650 to 1,300x10^9/L) were similar to those ending in abortion (median 900x10^9/L; range 600 to 1,300x10^9/L). However, platelet counts before pregnancy (median 850x10^9/L) were significantly higher as compared with the lowest platelet counts during pregnancy (median 510x10^9/L) (P=0.01). During the postpartum period platelet counts gradually returned to pre-pregnancy levels. No specific therapy was administred in nine pregnancies (seven abortions and two live births); in other eight pregnancies acetylsalicylic acid (ASA 100 mg/die) alone was used (three abortions and five live births). Our experience, in accordance with other authors, suggest that: a) women with ET have an increase risk of spontaneous abortion (59% compared with 15% expected in the general population) especially during the first trimester of pregnancy (80% of all abortions); this risk is not predictable by the preconception platelet count; b) the outcome of pregnancy in ET (live birth vs abortion) seems to be positively influenced by ASA; c) a significant and spontaneous decrease or normalization in platelet count during pregnancy in ET can be observed and this phenomenon may be related to the placental/fetal production of interferon like substances. The outcome and management of pregnancy in young women with ET is an increasing problem. On the basis of our findings and of the literature data, we found that large, multicentric and prospective studies are necessary in order to establish the best conduct and the optimal therapeutic approach in this particular subgroup of patients with CMD.

PO 41
Administration of GP IIB/IIIA Inhibitors Reduces Subacute Stent Thrombosis in Patients Affected by Cancer and Acute Coronary Syndromes

G SANGIORGI [1], F PIOVELLA [2], K GARRATT [4], D DE TOMA [3], M BARONE [2], M MEDDA [1], S BALANESCU [1], S CASTELVECCHIO [1], L INGLESE [1]*
[1]Cardiac Catheterization Laboratory, [3]Department of Oncology, Istituto Policlinico San Donato, University of Milan, [2]Thromboembolism Unit, IRCCS Policlinico San Matteo, Pavia, Italy; [4]Department of Cardiovascular Diseases, Mayo Clinic and Foundation, Rochester, MN USA

From different research investigations it appears that cancer not only activate coagulation systems, inducing a venous thrombophilic state, but also affects primary hemostasis which may cause arterial thrombosis in standard population cohorts. In particular, it has been demonstrated in vitro that tumor cells, through the release of ADP, cathepsin B-like cysteine proteinase, and PCA/PAA may trigger platelet aggregation directly (Grignani G. et al, Blood, 1988). Due to increase survival in patients affected by malignancies, the cardiologists may observe more patients with acute coronary syndromes and cancer for the increase of patient number suffering from both diseases. In addition, it is well known that those patients may benefit more from percutaneous coronary intervention (PCI) than surgery (due to the severe decrease in immuno-system defenses during CABG). Since pts affected malignancies show an hyper-coagulable/aggregation state, we hypothesized that patients affected by cancer and undergoing PCI for acute myocardial infarction (AMI) may benefit from the administration of glycoprotein IIb/IIIa inhibitors in order to reduce the risk of thrombotic complications. In our study, patients affected by cancer and presenting with AMI were submitted to PCI and coronary stent placement for the treatment of the culprit lesion. Patients were randomized either to 0.25mg/kg bolus followed by continuous infusion of 10μg/min of GPIIb/IIIa inhibitor abciximab (ReoPro, CentoCor BV, Leiden, Netherlands) or to standard therapy with heparin (100 units/kg) adjusted to achieve an activated thromboplastin time between 2 and 2.5 times normal. TIMI flow score at the end of the procedure, subacute stent thrombosis (thrombosis of the stented segment within 48 hrs from PCI), and major and minor bleeding were assessed. **Results**: A total of twelve patients (7 males and 4 females, 52±6yrs) presenting with AMI (8 anterior, 4 inferior) were evaluated. Five patients (3 affected by lung cancer, 2 affected by breast cancer) were treated with standard therapy (group A) and seven patients (2 affected by lung cancer, 1 by gastric cancer, 2 by breast cancer, and 1 by acute leukemia) with abciximab (group B) during PCI. No differences in age, cardiac risk factors and left ventricular ejection fraction were detected between the two groups at the time of enrollment. No differences in the number and length of stents were detected in the two study groups. Procedural technical success was obtained in all patients. No differences in TIMI score at the end of the procedure were present in the two groups. In group A, subacute thrombosis of the stent requiring a new emergency rescue PCI occurred in all patients. No stent thrombosis was detected in patiens treated by abciximab ($p<0.0001$). No major or minor bleedings occurred in the two study groups (p=ns). **Conclusions**: Administration of GP IIb/IIIa inhibitors during PCI is effective in reducing the rate of thrombotic complications in patients affected by malignancies undergoing PCI for acute myocardial infarction. Further larger clinical studies are needed to determine the long-term clinical benefit with this class of drugs in patients affected by malignancies and coronary atherosclerotic disease.

PO 42
The Risk of Recurrence After a First Episode of Venous Thromboembolism in Cancer Patients

B COSMI, C LEGNANI, S COCCHERI, G PALARETI*
Cardiovascular Department, Division of Angiology, S.Orsola–Malpighi Hospital, University of Bologna, Bologna, Italy

Background: The optimal duration of oral anticoagulant therapy (OAT) after a first episode of venous thromboembolism (VTE) in cancer patients is uncertain. OAT prolongation may be recommended until the disease is considered active or in case of chemotherapy. **Aim of the study**: To evaluate the recurrence rate after a first episode of VTE and OAT withdrawal in cancer patients. **Experimental design**: Prospective cohort study. **Patients & Methods**: We evaluated two cohorts of patients with a first objectively documented episode of deep vein thrombosis (DVT) and/or pulmonary embolism (PE). All patients received an initial course of heparin or low molecular weight heparin followed by OAT. In the first cohort, OAT was withdrawn at the discretion of the attending physician. In the second cohort, OAT was discontinued when the disease was considered eradicated by the oncologist on clinical and instrumental grounds and no chemotherapy was planned. Clinical follow-up was performed at 3, 9, 15 and 21 months after OAT withdrawal. Recurrence was diagnosed by compression ultrasound in case of DVT symptoms and non- or partial compressibility of a previously compressible venous segment. PE recurrence was diagnosed on the basis of V/Q scan. **Results**: In the first cohort, 38 patients (M/F: 15/23, mean age: 71; range: 34-88) were evaluated. Cancer site was prostate (4), breast (12), gastrointestinal (7), haematological (7), other (8). Twelve patients developed VTE after surgery performed to eradicate the cancer, 3 during chemotherapy and 1 during tamoxifen treatment for breast cancer. The mean duration of OAT was: 6 months, range 3-28. Thirteen patients developed recurrent VTE during a total 55.2 patient/years (pt/y) follow-up (23.5%pt/y). In the second cohort, 36 patients (M/F: 20/16, mean age: 62; range: 37-87) were evaluated. Cancer site was prostate (8), breast (9), gastrointestinal (3), lung (4), haematological (4), other (8). Fifteen patients developed VTE after surgery performed to eradicate the cancer, 13 during chemotherapy and 2 during tamoxifen treatment for breast cancer. The mean duration of OAT was: 10 months, range 1-40. OAT was withdrawn in 24 patients. OAT was prolonged in 12 patients for metastatic disease (6) and planned chemotherapy (6). In a total follow-up of 15.6 pt/y, only one patient developed recurrent VTE after OAT withdrawal (6.4%pt/y). **Conclusions**: The rate of recurrence in cancer patients after a first episode of VTE is low when OAT is withdrawn only in patients in whom the disease is considered to be clinically and instrumentally eradicated.

PO 43
Adverse Interactions between Continuous Infusion of 5-Fluorouracil (5-FU) Based Chemotherapy and Warfarin Inducing Prothrombin Time Abnormalities

G MASCI, PA ZUCALI, B SARINA, M MAGAGNOLI, L CASTAGNA, M FALLINI, C CARNAGHI, A SANTORO
Department of Medical Oncology and Hematology ; Istituto Clinico Humanitas, Rozzano (Milan), Italy

Background: The daily use of anticoagulant prophylaxis in patients with central venous catheter (CVC) had established role against thrombotic events, with a very low hemorragic risk. We retrospectively examined the incidence of bleeeding and International Normalized Ratio (INR) alteration in gastrointestinal cancer patients treated in our institution with continuous 5-FU infusion based chemotherapy. **Materials & Methods**: Between July 1999 and August 2001, 70 consecutive cancer patients were evaluated. The median age was 47 (range 34-78 y). Fifty-eight pts were affected by colon cancer, 6 by gastric cancer, 3 by pancreatic cancer, 2 by gallbladder carcinoma and 1 by esophageal cancer. Thirty-four patients had liver metastasis. Sixty-four patients had CVC Groshong tipy and 6 a port-a-cath. All patients received warfarin 1 mg/daily as prophylaxis against catheter-associated thrombosis. **Results**: INR alteration occured in 34% (24/70) of patients during chemotherapy administration. Minor bleeding (epistaxis and hematuria) was observed in 6/70 pts and was not correlated with risk of death or hospitalization. In all but one pts the INR was abnormal. Of the 24 pts with INR abnormalities, 10 had liver metastasis. No correlation was found between liver metastasis and INR alteration or bleeding. No statistical significative differences was observed between pts with or without liver metastasis, in terms of bleeding or INR alteration. None of the 70 patients receiving warfarin had catheter–associated thrombosis. **Conclusions**: A high incidence of INR abnormalities was observed in our cohort of cancer patients treated with 5-FU and warfarin. The nature and the extent of this interaction should be elucidated by a prospective study. Until that time regular monitoring of the prothrombin time in these patients is recommended.

PO 44
Incidence of Newly Diagnosed Cancer after Three Months or One Year of Oral Anticoagulation for a First Episode of Idiopathic Venous Thromboembolism

MR TALIANI, G AGNELLI, P PRANDONI, C BECATTINI, M MOIA, M BAZZAN, C TOMASI, C GUAZZALOCA, A BERTOLDI, W AGENO, GB AMBROSIO, R SALVI, R POGGIO, M SILINGARDI, F PORRO, P ZONZIN, D IMBERTI, F CASAZZA, E POGLIANI, L RIA, F PIOVELLA, D DE LUCIA, FOR THE WARFARIN OPTIMAL DURATION ITALIAN TRIAL INVESTIGATORS*

Background: A number of studies reported the association between idiopathic venous thromboembolism (VTE) and subsequent diagnosis of cancer. The risk of newly diagnosed cancer has been reported to be higher in patients with VTE treated with oral anticoagulants (OA) for six weeks than in patients treated for six months. **Aim of the study**: To evaluate, in a multicenter prospective randomized study, if one-year anticoagulation reduces the risk of newly diagnosed cancer in patients with idiopathic VTE with respect to three-month anticoagulation. **Methods**: Patients with a first episode of VTE not associated with temporary risk factors (i.e. surgery, trauma, oral contraceptives, etc.) or persistent risk factors (known cancer and thrombophilia) were included in the study. After three months of oral anticoagulation (INR: 2 to 3), patients were randomized to withdraw anticoagulation or to continue it for 9 additional months. Newly diagnosed cancer was assessed by follow-up visits scheduled every three months for the first year and every 6 months for the following years after randomization. **Results**: 419 patients (267 presenting with DVT and 152 with PE, 53% males; age 65 years) were enrolled in the study at 20 Italian hospitals. During a mean follow up of 45.7 months, newly diagnosed cancer occurred in 25 patients (6.0%):11 out of 206 patients (5.3%) treated with OA for 3 months and 14 out of 213 patients (6.6%) treated for 12 months (RR=0.81, 95% CI 0.37-1.74). Cancer sites were urogenital tract (7 patients), respiratory tract (5), gastrointestinal system (5), breast (5), hemopoietic system (3). No difference in the incidence of death related to cancer was found between the two groups. **Conclusions**: In patients with idiopathic VTE one-year anticoagulation does not have a protective effect on the development of newly diagnosed cancer with respect to three-month anticoagulation.

PO 45
Pulmonary Artery Sarcoma (Angiosarcoma) Mimicking Chronic Major Vessel Thromboembolic Pulmonary Hypertensive Disease (CTPH)

F PIOVELLA [1], P FEDULLO [3], M BARONE [1], C PORTA [2], S SERAFINI [1], S FERRARI [2], A NATALIZI [1], L LIBRE' [1], M DANOVA [2]*

[1]Servizio Malattie Tromboemboliche, [2]Medicina Interna ed Oncologia medica, IRCCS Policlinico San Matteo, Pavia, Italy; [3]Pulmonary and Critical Care Division, Department of Medicine, University of California at San Diego Medical Center, La Jolla, CA, USA.

A 53-year-old male was referred to our Thromboembolism Unit for evaluation of severe pulmonary hypertension presumed to be secondary to chronic pulmonary thromboemboli. Patient was well until two years before admission when he complained of vague intermittent left-sided chest pain. No leg swelling was reported, nor a prior history of venous thromboembolism. Spiral CT scan revealed a filling defect obstructing the left pulmonary artery and the majority of the right pulmonary artery. Perfusion lung scan demonstrated absence of blood flow to the entire left lung and to the anterior and apical segments of the upper lobe of the right lung. Pulmonary angiography demonstrated complete obstruction of the left pulmonary artery with only a small channel providing blood flow to the right lung. The patient was referred for thromboendarterectomy. On physical examination, the patient showed most of the signs and symptoms characteristic of CTPH. Uncommon digital clubbing, which had developed during the 2 to 3 months before admission, was present. Cardiac catheterization showed pulmonary artery pressure (PAP) 90/25 mm Hg, mean 48 mm Hg. Cardiac output (CO) was 1.72 L/min. Pulmonary vascular resistance (PVR) was 2,046 dyne/cm^2. Patient underwent pulmonary artery exploration. A large mass completely filling the left pulmonary artery and the proximal right pulmonary artery was encountered. The mass was successfully resected. Pathologic examination of the tissue was consistent with a spindle cell sarcoma. Postoperative hemodynamics disclosed PAP= 30/40 mm Hg, mean 19 mm Hg, CO= 3.97 L/min, and PVR= 128 dyne/cm^2. Patient's functional status improved from NYHA class III to class I. Our patient had an uneventful postoperative recovery. Two years later he died from massive bleeding due to the rupture of the inferior vena cava, the site where the tumour originated.

PO 46
Cardiac Thrombus Associated to Angiosarcoma

C ROTHSCHILD, CM MASSUMOTO*
Hospital Santa Paula/ Centro de Hemoterapia São Lucas, São Paulo, Brazil

Primary cardiac angiosarcoma is a rare tumour, although it is the most commom of primary cardiac malignancies. Rarely it can be accompanied by a cardiac thrombus, which represents a major risk factor for embolic events. The authors describe the case of a 48-year-old man who had the diagnosis of a primary cardiac angiosarcoma with pulmonary metastasis. As the echocardiogram had showed two right atrial masses and it had not been possible to perform a biopsy at that time, anticoagulation was started in order to avoid an embolism. After some months of chemotherapy, the patient underwent a surgical resection of the cardiac masses, one of which was in fact a thrombus. Anticoagulation has been maintained until now, under close monitoring and there were no bleeding nor thromboembolic episodes. A prophylactic anticoagulation may be useful in preventing fatal embolism in patients with cardiac tumours.

PO 47
Femoral Venous Thrombosis in Two Patients with Diffuse Large Cell Lymphoma

C ROTHSCHILD, HA LOTERIO*
Faculdade de Medicina de Jundiaí, São Paulo, Brazil

One of the mechanisms by which a malignancy can cause thromboembolism is vascular compression due to a mass. Here are reported the cases of two patients with diffuse large cell lymphoma who developed femoral venous thrombosis associated to inguinal enlarged lymph nodes. The first one was a 41-year-old man who had already completed six cycles of chemotherapy and presented a new lymph node enlargement with thrombosis. The other was a 68-year-old man who was admitted with the clinical picture of thrombosis due to femoral vein compression. Both patients started anticoagulation, which was maintained and carefully monitored during all antineoplastic treatment. There were no bleeding episodes related to antithrombotic therapy. Local vascular compression can contribute to venous thrombosis and its complications, sometimes fatal. This may be prevented by the use of antithrombotic agents, which close monitoring can avoid bleeding complications.

PO 48
Central Venous Line Related Thrombosis in Children with Acute Lymphoblastic Leukemia: A Prospective Study

P SARACCO[1], L FARINASSO[1], TM GAJNO[2], A VALORI[3], MF CAMPAGNOLI[1], C ALLIAUDI[1], N FERRERO[4], L CORDERO DI MONTEZEMOLO[1], U RAMENGHI[1]*
[4]Servizio Trasfusionale, Azienda OIRM-S. Anna, [1]Divisione di Ematologia Pediatrica, Università di Torino, [2]UOA Neuroradiologia, [3]UOA Cardiochirurgia, Turin, Italy

The exact incidence of central venous line (CVL) related deep venous thrombosis (DVT) in children with cancer is not known, but surely underestimated. Choice of diagnostic radiographic test, particularly to detect asymptomatic DVT, has directly influenced studies results so far. Non invasive testing as ultrasound (US) and lineograms fail to diagnose DVT in the central intrathoracic veins (CIV), and bilateral upper limb venography remains the gold standard diagnostic test, but is not easily performed in children. Spiral computed tomography (CT) is a non invasive and valid alternative to venography and may be used to detect and monitor both symptomatic and asymptomatic persistent vascular CVL related thrombosis or occlusion (defined as narrowing, obstruction or filling defects of DV system with or without collateral veins). Aim of this ongoing prospective study is to detect the incidence of symptomatic and asymptomatic CVL related DVT, by using CT and US, in a cohort of children with acute lymphoblastic leukemia (ALL) consecutively diagnosed since december 1999 and with newly inserted CVL. Spiral CT (Siemens Somaton Plus and Magic View software for three dimensional reconstruction of angiograms) is performed at various time from CVL insertion (30-60 days or end of chemotherapy induction, 6 months or at maintenance treatment, at the stop of therapy or at CVL removal and thereafter in case of detected occlusion). Twenty-three children (age range 14 mo.-15 yrs), treated according to AIEOP ALL 95 and 2000 protocols (8 and 15 respectively) are being studied: in all cases the CVL insertion technique was venous cut-down, in over 70 % of cases via right Jugular vein and all performed standard thromboprophylaxis with unfractionated heparin (UH) CVL flushes.All children were screened for prothrombotic genetic factors (Leiden, 20210, MTHFR, lp(A)). The first CT scan detected DVT-occlusion (jugular and CIV) in 12 out of 23 (52%): of these only 5 had symptoms of suspected CVL obstruction and 1 subsequently developed a superior vena cava syndrome (CVL with unproperly large lumen). This study confirms the significant incidence of CVL related DVT or occlusion, in children with ALL despite regular UH CVL flushes prophylaxis and validates the use of spiral CT for detection and monitoring of asymptomatic DVT. Randomized trials to check a different prophylactic anticoagulation or other prevention approach are urgently needed in these patients.

PO 49
High Dose Methotrexate in Children with Acute Lymphoblastic Leukemia: Hyperhomocysteinemia, Thrombotic Risk and Toxicity

P SARACCO, P ANGELINI, L FARINASSO, E BARISONE, MF CAMPAGNOLI, C ALLIAUDI, F ALTARE, F BONETTI, E MADON*
Divisione di Ematologia, Azienda Ospedaliera OIRM-Sant'Anna, Turin, Italy

Methotrexate (MTX) is an antifolate chemotherapeutic drug and toxicity includes mucositis and myelosuppression. It has been postulated that MTX sensitivity varies with genetic variability in folate- metabolizing enzymes. A central folate metabolism enzyme is methylentetrahydrofolate reductase (MTHFR) which converts homocysteine to methionine. A common (10-12% of caucasian and asian population) MTHFR polymorphism (C6771T) results in reduced activity (30% in homozygous TT and 60% in heterozygotes CT variant) which causes an accumulation of homocysteine, a protrombotic risk factor. The effectiveness of MTX is attributable to its role as inhibitor of dihydrofolate reductase and other folate enzymes as MTHFR, and it lowers folate levels. In this study, we have evaluated levels of homocysteinemia (by HPLC method) and risk for vascular occlusion as well as toxicity during high dose MTX treatment (3 g/sqm 24 hrs infusion followed by leucovorin rescue, for a total of 4 courses) among 21 children (age range 14 m-15 y) with acute lymphoblastic leukemia (ALL) consecutively diagnosed since september 2000 at our institution , and treated according to AIEOP 2000 protocol. Aim of the study was to investigate differences in outcomes (hyperomocysteinemia and risk of thrombosis, mucositis and hematological toxicity measured by OMS score, and MTX serum levels) by MTHFR genotype comparison: CT (12 out of 21 patients, 57%) and TT (2 out of 21, 9%) genotypes (total 14 patients) versus CC genotype (7 patients, 33%). Results: mean homocysteinemia increased significantly after first course MTX compared to basal in all patients; hematological toxicity (score 3-4 by OMS grading) was present only in the CT/TT genotypes and persisted in the subsequent courses; mucositis (score 3-4) was evident in 43% of CT/TT and in 28% of normal variant; all CC patients showed a normal MTX clearance, while 36% of CT/TT patients had persistent MTX high serum levels requiring further rescue. In 2 patients with CT/TT genotype and homocysteinemia over 30 μM a thrombotic event occurred during MTX treatment (9%). The study confirms relationship between the CT/TT MTHFR variant and MTX toxicity as recently described (Ulrich et al., Blood 2001) as well as the further risk of vascular disease during MTX treatment in children with ALL. Tailored prophylaxis both for toxicity and thrombotic risk (as protracted or increased leucovorin rescue, oral glutamine administration or anti-coagulation) might be helpful in ALL patients with CT/TT genotype.

PO 50
Pulmonary Thromboembolism as Presentation of Acute Myeloid Leukemia, Successfully Treated with Enoxaparin

D VALLISA, D IMBERTI, R BERTE', G CIVARDI, C MORONI, A LAZZARO, L CAVANNA*
Medical Oncology and Ematology Unit, Civic Hospital, Piacenza, Italy

Clinical case: On December 2000 a Caucasian 27 years-old man was referred to our Department for an ongoing history of deep vein thrombosis that began one month before with thrombosis of left subclavian vein, thereafter the patient developed deep vein thrombosis of left leg. At the admission the patient showed swelling of the left leg and dispnea; ventiloperfusion lung scan revealed bilateral pulmonary embolism while deep vein thrombosis of the left leg was confirmed by echocolordoppler. Laboratory evaluation allowed us to disclose absolute neutropenia with mild leucopenia, peripheral blood smear showed circulating blasts (4%). Platelet count and coagulative parameters were in normal range except high increase of fibrin degradation products. Suddenly the patient underwent bone marrow evaluation that allowed us to diagnose acute myeloid leukemia M1 with blasts expressing CD34, CD7, CD33 and MPO. Therefore an antracycline containing chemiotherapic regimen was started together with enoxaparin 10,000 UI twice a day subcutaneously (patient body weight: 110 kg). Dispnea and swelling of the leg disappeared. When platelet count was below 20,000/μl enoxaparin was reduced to 10,000 UI once a day and then increased to 8,000 UI twice a day when platelets overcame 50,000/μl. The same enoxaparin schedule was applied during the second cytostatic reinduction cycle (the patient did not reach complete response with the first cycle but he did with the second one). Enoxaparin treatment was continued also during consolidation cycles and during mobilization of peripheral blood stem cells that reached a good harvest. On July 2001, the patient was sent to another center for allografting procedure evaluation and the colleagues substituted enoxaparin with warfarin. Three weeks later the patient developed hematuria with typical lumbar colic pain and then left leg hematoma with a consequent suspension of oral anticoagulant. **Conclusions**: Enoxaparin revealed to be efficacious and safe in the management of a patient affected by acute myelod leukemia complicated by deep vein thrombosis with pulmonary embolism. As a matter of fact enoxaparin cured acute vein thrombosis, prevented recurrency and did not cause any hemorragic complication despite prolonged severe piastrinopenia.

PO 51
Recurrent Venous Thromboembolism and Bleeding Complications During Anticoagulant Treatment in Patients with Cancer and Venous Thrombosis

P PRANDONI, AWA LENSING, A PICCIOLI, F NOVENTA, P BAGATELLA, E BERNARDI, B GIROLAMI, A MARCHIORI, P SABBION, P SIMIONI, MH PRINS, A GIROLAMI*
Department of Medical and Surgical Sciences, University of Padova, Italy;
Academic Medical Center, University of Amsterdam, The Netherlands

A small proportion of patients with deep-vein thrombosis (DVT) develops recurrent venous thromboembolic (VTE) complications or bleeding during anticoagulant treatment. These complications may occur more frequently if such patients have concomitant cancer. Little is known whether the perceived higher risks for recurrent VTE and bleeding during anticoagulation apply to all patients with cancer or to certain subtypes only. Consecutive outpatients with confirmed symptomatic DVT with or without cancer participated in the study. Type and stage of cancer were classified as severe, moderately severe, or less severe. Heparinization and subsequent oral anticoagulation were given in therapeutic dosages and duration of treatment depended on the presence of risk factors. Patients were prospectively followed for a maximum of one year to document the incidence of recurrent VTE complications and bleeding, and hazard ratios (HR) were obtained. Patients were censored for the analysis at the time of cessation of anticoagulant treatment. Of the 842 included patients, 181 had known cancer at entry. Cancer was severe in 37.6%, moderately severe in 22.1%, and less severe in 40.3% of patients. The 12-month cumulative incidence of major bleeding was 12.4% (95% CI: 6.6-18.2%) in patients with cancer and 5.0% (95% CI: 2.5-7.5%) in patients without cancer, for a HR of 2.2 (95% CI: 1.2-4.1; p=0.015). Recurrence and bleeding were both related to cancer severity but could not be explained by sub- or over-coagulation. Cancer patients with DVT are more likely to develop recurrent thromboembolic complications and major bleeding than those without malignancy. These risks increase with cancer severity. Optimization of monitoring procedures for anticoagulant therapy has the potential to improve outcome in only a small subset of patients.

PO 52
Feasibility and Safety of Low-Dose Warfarin Prophylaxis of VTE in Different Categories of Advanced Cancer Patients

*D FAGNANI, P TAGLIABUE, P POZZI, A FERRARIO, C CIMMINIELLO**
Servizio di Oncologia, Dipartimento di Medicina, Ospedale Civile di Vimercate, Vimercate, Italy

Cancer itself is known to be one of the most potent risk factors of venous thromboembolism (VTE). Moreover advanced stages of disease, chemotherapy and the presence of central venous lines are additional oncologic factors increasing the risk of VTE. Levine et al. (Lancet 1994) demonstrated that low-dose warfarin is an effective prophylactic regimen allowing a significant reduction of symptomatic VTE in women affected by advanced breast cancer during chemotherapy. Aim of the present observation was to evaluate whether the same warfarin schedule proposed by Levine - that is 1 mg warfarin daily for the first 6 weeks then targeting INR between 1.3 and 1.9 - is feasible and safe also in patients suffering from advanced malignancies other than breast cancer and at high risk of VTE because the contemporary treatment with chemotherapy and the carrying of central venous lines. Fifty-two patients, mean age 62.4 (median 63 yrs), were evaluated, all affected by advanced (M+) disease: 66% of them suffered from colorectal cancer, 14% from breast cancer, 12% from pancreatic cancer and 8% from stomach cancer. All patients were receiving chemotherapy and were carriers of central venous lines. The mean duration of oral anticoagulant treatment was 8.2 months (median 6.5 months) The occurrence of symptomatic (objectively confirmed) VTE events (one PE and two DVTs) was observed in 3 patients (5.8%) while 2 episodes of superficial venous thrombosis occurred in one additional patient at the site of central venous accesses. It is also to underline that all the 3 VTE patients suffered from a recurrence of VTE during secondary prophylaxis with larger doses of warfarin. Only one episode of GI bleeding was noticed in a treated patient while his INR value was in the target range but he was also assuming NSAIDs. These preliminary results seem to indicate that warfarin prophylaxis according to Levine is feasible and safe also in cancer patients with advanced disease other than breast cancer but the optimal intensity of oral anticoagulation should be assessed in specific ad hoc designed studies owing the fact that there seems to exist cancer subjects highly prone to thrombosis.

PO 53
Comparison of In-Patient Admission Vs Nurse Led Ambulatory Management of DVT: Incidence of Cancer at 6 Months

S RHODES, S BOND, N PEMBERTON, ES GREEN, P ROSE, R BROWN*
Departments of Haematology and Audit, Swindon, Warwick and Walsgrave, United Kingdom

In the United Kingdom there is an increasing role for clinical nurse specialists (CNS) to provide assessment and subsequent management of patients presenting with deep vein thrombosis (DVT). We compared three different services in respect of diagnosis and subsequent development of malignancy. Six hundred and eighty-four (684) patients with proven DVT with a follow-up of 6 months were screened for subsequent malignancies from histology computerised records, hospital notes and patient administration systems where in-patient episodes occurred. At site A with CNS assessment only, of 198 patients 39 (20%) had an underlying malignancy recorded at diagnosis and 3 patients subsequently developed a malignancy post DVT, 2 with metastatic lung cancer may have been identified earlier. At site B with initial review by junior medical staff followed by CNS ambulatory DVT management, of 237 patients 27 (11%) had a malignancy recorded at diagnosis with 6 subsequent malignancies. Only 2 of these were not under investigation for suspected malignancy at the time of DVT presentation (1 Ca colon, 1 Ca breast). At site C with traditional in-patient management (review by 3 or more medical staff) of 251 patients 45 (18%) had a malignancy recorded at diagnosis with 3 subsequently developing malignancy. In-patient investigations included more blood, radiological and invasive procedures, some of which were deemed inappropriate. No benefit from medical admission was identified and we have not shown an increased risk of CNS management in respect of assessment and identification of malignancy. We have introduced a common algorithm to try and identify patients in need of additional investigations. This study is ongoing and is being implemented by CNS in preference to medical staff.

Author Index

Haemostasis 2001;31(suppl. 1)